Diagnosing Dental and Orofacial Pain:
A Clinical Manual

Dedication

To Judy-Ann and Lisa
For patience and understanding.

Diagnosing Dental and Orofacial Pain: A Clinical Manual

Edited by

Alex J. Moule

M. Lamar Hicks

WILEY Blackwell

Library of Congress Cataloging-in-Publication Data

Names: Moule, A. J. (Alex J.), editor. | Hicks, M. Lamar, editor.
Title: Diagnosing dental and orofacial pain : a clinical manual / edited by
Alex J. Moule, M. Lamar Hicks.
Description: Chichester, West Sussex, UK ; Ames, Iowa : John Wiley & Sons, Inc., 2017. |
Includes bibliographical references and index.
Identifiers: LCCN 2016022484 (print) | LCCN 2016023021 (ebook) | ISBN 9781118925003 (pbk.) |
ISBN 9781118924990 (pdf) | ISBN 9781118924983 (epub)
Subjects: | MESH: Facial Pain–diagnosis | Toothache–diagnosis
Classification: LCC RK322 (print) | LCC RK322 (ebook) | NLM WU 140 |
DDC 617.5/2–dc23
LC record available at https://lccn.loc.gov/2016022484

A catalogue record for this book is available from the British Library.

Wiley also publishes its books in a variety of electronic formats. Some content that appears in print may not be available in electronic books.

1   2017

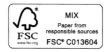

Contents

Contributors

Vishal R. Aggarwal
Clinical Associate Professor in Acute Dental Care
    and Chronic Pain
School of Dentistry, Faculty of Medicine and Health
University of Leeds
Leeds, UK

Tareq Al Ali
Faculty of Dentistry
Kuwait University
Kuwait

Michael J. Apicella
Rohde Dental Clinic
Fort Bragg, NC, USA

Scott Cook
Director
The Headache, Neck and Jaw Clinic
(formerly Body Mechanics Physiotherapy)
Brisbane, QLD, Australia

Dr Kerryn Green
Consultant Neurologist
Royal Brisbane and Women's Hospital
Senior Lecturer
University of Queensland
Brisbane, QLD, Australia

M. Lamar Hicks
Endodontics Division
University of Maryland Dental School
Baltimore, MD, USA

Iven Klineberg
Professor and Head of Prosthodontics
University of Sydney
Jaw Function and Orofacial Pain Research Unit
Westmead Hospital Centre of Oral Health
Westmead, NSW, Australia

Unni Krishnan
School of Dentistry
University of Queensland
Brisbane, Australia

David Mock
Professor and Dean Emeritus
Oral Medicine/Oral Pathology
University of Toronto
Toronto, ON, Canada

Alex J. Moule
School of Dentistry
University of Queensland
Brisbane, QLD, Australia

Chris Moule
Prosthodontist
Private Practice
Clinical Educator
Faculty of Dentistry
University of Sydney
Sydney, NSW, Australia

Mark Paine
Consultant Neurologist/Neuro-ophthalmologist
Alexandra Neurology
Brisbane, QLD, Australia

E. Russell Vickers
Oral and Maxillofacial Surgeon
University of Sydney Medical School
Sydney, NSW, Australia

Andrew D. Wolvin
Department of Communication
University of Maryland
College Park, MD, USA

ILLUSTRATIONS
Jerry Liu
Jerry Liu Design and Photography
Brisbane, QLD, Australia

Acknowledgments

I must acknowledge the many clinicians, colleagues, authors and lecturers who have assisted with this manual over so many years. It has been over twenty years in the making. Much of the information in it has been gleaned from over forty years of clinical practice treating patients presenting with orofacial pain. The source of information is often clouded by time, and my thanks must go to the countless colleagues with whom I have discussed the management of patients.

My thanks also to the many authors who have contributed to this project, without whom this manual would never had been written, and to many friends and family who willed it to completion. I thank my colleagues at the Faculty of Dentistry, Kuwait University, for their support and friendship as I worked on this manuscript.

Thank you Jerry Liu for the illustrations, and a heartfelt thanks to my co-editor, Lamar Hicks, who reviewed chapter after chapter and brought them all to life. My love and thanks to my wife, Judy-Ann, and my sons and daughter who have all travelled this long editorial journey with me.

Alex J. Moule

About the Companion Website

This book is accompanied by a companion website:

www.wiley.com/go/moule/dental_and_orofacial_pain

The website includes:

- Case studies that serve as examples for several chapters
- 22 videos that are cited throughout the book
- Clinical Pain Inventory Form
- Personal Pain Plan by the Australian Pain Management Association (APMA).

Chapter 1

Introduction

Alex J. Moule and M. Lamar Hicks

Introduction

Clinicians are called upon to diagnose orofacial pain on a daily basis. For the most part, diagnosis is a routine procedure which is accomplished without too much difficulty. Most painful conditions follow certain predictable patterns and exhibit specific signs and symptoms which, when observed, make diagnosis a relatively easy task to perform. Patients do present, however, where diagnosis is especially difficult and where pain patterns do not follow recognized norms. Many of these difficult cases can have unsatisfactory outcomes for both patients and practitioners.

There are numerous textbooks that deal with pain diagnosis. Most of these provide a comprehensive review of the signs, symptoms and pathology associated with the various conditions that can cause facial pain. Few deal with the actual process of diagnosing orofacial pain, and even fewer deal in any detail with the specific questions and tests that are required to establish a diagnosis for each condition.

This manual addresses some of the difficulties in assessing patients with orofacial pain by *focusing on the questions that need to be asked* and *analyzing responses of patients to these questions*. This is in contrast to just describing the various painful conditions. Particular attention is paid to the *meaning of descriptors* patients use when describing pain.

From a practical point of view, the initial task for a practitioner in assessing a patient with orofacial pain is a reasonably simple process: to establish whether the patient has a dental pain problem, a treatable non-dental pain problem, or a pain problem that requires referral to a dental or medical specialist. Once this broad sorting is carried out, more specific diagnosis and treatment planning can take place for each condition. To place the patient into one of these categories is often relatively uncomplicated. Nevertheless, mistakes often occur because *practitioners jump to conclusions before assessing all of the facts*, and because insufficient information is gathered before a diagnosis is made. Thus, when diagnosing pain, *history is more important than testing*. Indeed, it is the history that dictates the tests to perform. History is obtained by asking appropriate questions. Diagnosis is based on:

- Observing the patient (*"What should I look for?"*)
- Knowing the questions to ask (*"What should I ask?"*)
- Analyzing the answers received (*"What does this answer mean?" "What else do I need to know?"*)
- Performing appropriate tests
- Applying all this information to the task of identifying the problem.

When diagnosing pain, there are two broad categories of questions that the clinician must be able to use. The first category is a series of general sorting or screening questions that elicit a broad picture of the pain profile. These form the basis for asking the second category of questions, which are *specific screening questions* used for a particular pain state (e.g. dental pain, muscle pain, trigeminal neuralgia, cluster headache). Unless a practitioner is aware of the specific questions that relate to the different pain states, an accurate diagnosis of challenging pain cases is difficult or impossible to make.

Mistakes in diagnosis are often made when clinicians approach the diagnosis too quickly without first analyzing the patient's responses to questions, and when attempts are made to *make the facts fit a diagnosis* rather than *make the diagnosis fit the facts*.

Diagnosing Dental and Orofacial Pain: A Clinical Manual, First Edition. Edited by Alex J. Moule and M. Lamar Hicks.
© 2017 John Wiley & Sons, Ltd. Published 2017 by John Wiley & Sons, Ltd.
Companion website: www.wiley.com/go/moule/dental_and_orofacial_pain

When confronted with any diagnostic situation it is helpful to remember a "golden rule":

If it doesn't add up, it doesn't add up.

When confronted with any diagnostic situation that does not add up, it is helpful to remember a second "golden rule":

If it doesn't add up, then review it again or refer.

Similarly, if confronted with any diagnostic situation that does not add up and does not respond to initial treatment, it is helpful to remember a third important rule:

Do not "walk" along teeth.

When confronted with a patient with a complex pain problem, great care should be taken not to keep trying to find a dental cause by treating one tooth after another in an attempt to relieve pain that may or may not be dental in origin. Before treatment is initiated, an accurate diagnosis must be established (Fig. 1-1).

In the following chapters, the causes of orofacial pain will be identified and explained and the diagnostic processes that are necessary to arrive at

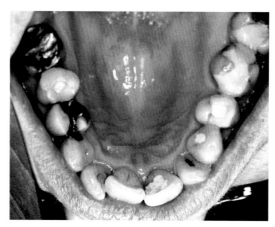

Fig. 1-1 A patient with non-dental pain who had multiple restorations and endodontic procedures in an unsuccessful attempt to relieve orofacial pain.

an accurate diagnosis will be discussed. Particular attention is placed on:

- How to record a pain profile
- How to listen to and observe a patient in pain
- How to analyze responses to questions
- How to formulate questions.

Specific screening questions are described for each pain condition. Short and long case reports are presented in the accompanying e-web material.

Chapter 2

The Art of Listening – Communicating Effectively with a Patient in Pain

Andrew D. Wolvin

Introduction

Good health care is a partnership between the patient and the clinician – and with the rest of a clinical team. The center of this partnership is effective communication. Research reinforces that *"communication between clinicians and patients has been recognized as an integral part of providing optimum patient care."*[1] This clinician–patient partnership should be built on a relationship of trust. It requires that the clinician be comforting, caring and encouraging, asking and answering questions, offering clear explanations, and listening and checking understanding.[2] Most patients who have orofacial pain seek advice first from a dentist. It is especially important with these patients to establish trust and develop good dentist–patient communication, which has been described as one that is purposeful: creating a good interpersonal relationship, exchanging information and deciding on the best course of treatment.[3] Not surprisingly, most of the focus in studies of dentist–patient communication has centered on dentists, with little attention to the communication needs of patients themselves. A national survey, for example, which asked dentists about their communication strategies[4] determined that good strategies that can be used include interpersonal communication, the teach-back method, patient-friendly materials and aids, the offering of assistance, and a patient-friendly practice. These communication techniques are what the dentist should say and/or do in interactions with patients.

However, since communication is a keystone of good patient care, it can be helpful to look more broadly at dentist–patient communication, not as dentist-centered, but as *listening-centered*. As the research stresses, communicating clinicians not only should utilize effective speaking skills, but also must engage in careful listening. Good clinical practice requires that you listen with your ears and your eyes to assess what you and the patient need to know, and what the patient already knows and wants to know.[5] It is important to start any interaction with good listening.[6] It is important to your diagnosis to know what the patient is experiencing and, to explore this, consider beginning your interaction with small talk that can help to establish a basic level of communication comfort. This often overlooked step is important for your patient to feel as much at ease as is possible in their interaction with you. This is challenging, of course, because if the patient has a significant orofacial pain problem, they will undoubtedly be apprehensive about what is wrong and what you will need to do to resolve the problem.

Beginning your interaction with small talk is time well spent, however, because you can learn a great deal about a patient's issue by listening perceptively to them in the beginning. Consider not starting out with the traditional *"How are you?"* greeting as a patient, understandably, cannot return the standard *"Fine, thanks"* response – thinking rather, *"I'm here for you to determine how I am!"* Instead, starting out with answerable questions such as: *"What is the temperature outside today?"* or *"How is the traffic out there?"* or *"You must be a Nationals fan?"* can help you establish rapport and in the process reduce your patient's anxiety.

Once you have provided a comforting opener, a question such as: *"What can I do for you today?"* establishes a good foundation to start your diagnosis. Listen closely then to what your patient tells you

Diagnosing Dental and Orofacial Pain: A Clinical Manual, First Edition. Edited by Alex J. Moule and M. Lamar Hicks.
© 2017 John Wiley & Sons, Ltd. Published 2017 by John Wiley & Sons, Ltd.
Companion website: www.wiley.com/go/moule/dental_and_orofacial_pain

about his/her issue. Ask the necessary follow-up questions to get the details you need. Most of your patients are not schooled in dental health, so you will need to probe further as to what is the problem. To effectively listen to your patients, you have to *ask all the relevant questions* to prompt the details you require to make an accurate diagnosis. These prompts are important. You do not want to run the risk of the *doorknob syndrome* where the patient remembers to tell the health care provider the *real issue* only as the consultation is coming to an end. Furthermore, you will want to check your understanding to be sure that what you heard is what the patient intended to communicate, echoing the patient's concerns by asking questions such as:

As I understand it, you've had this pain in the upper right side of your face for three days and it's getting worse…

When considering questioning, it may be helpful to remember the journalist's agenda: what, when, where, why and how, or more classically in pain diagnosis, the onset, duration, frequency, location, character, radiation, severity, the precipitating factors and the relieving factors all need to be addressed. How to phrase these questions and the relevance of the answers are the subjects of this manual.

At the same time, do not ignore the *visual channel*. Often, you can get a sense of a patient's level of pain from their nonverbal demeanor – facial grimaces, rigid posture, clutching the chair. Also note whether the nonverbal reaction is or is not consistent with the verbal responses you are hearing. A patient might tell you that their pain level is a 2 on a 10-point linear analogue scale, but their facial tension might well register an 8, or vice versa. Also, research on nonverbal communication suggests that as much as 55% of the emotional component of a message is communicated through the face alone, because individuals are not skilled at controlling their facial expression (and eye behavior), especially when in pain.[7] Additionally, pay particular attention to the manner in which a patient describes the location of their pain, as gestures and facial expression are often diagnostic for a given pain cause.

As your patient tells you about their orofacial pain problem, it is important to *be there as a listener*. You will want to attend to their narrative and to concentrate fully on what they have to say. In addition to your clinical observation procedures, do not be afraid to be emotionally empathetic and understanding to your patient as well. It is, of course, tempting in many situations to go straight to a diagnosis just as a patient launches into a description of an issue (after all, you will have heard this hundreds of times before). One study revealed that medical professionals tend to start directing the diagnostic discussion as early as 23 seconds into the intake interview,[8] before a patient has had time to explain their problem. Such premature diagnosis can lead you astray. You want to be sure you have heard the *full story* from your patient's perspective before coming to a conclusion, and to be aware that *a diagnosis must fit the facts*. It is risky to try to make the facts fit a diagnosis.

Listening to your patient's perspective is the key to being a responsive communicator. Once you have obtained all the details you need, your communication goal is then to explain fully what their problem is, and what course of treatment will resolve the problem. This can be a challenge, because most patients tend to be highly anxious, so they may not fully comprehend what you are recommending. Adding to the communication difficulty may be the level of *dental literacy* your patient has and that many patients often have turned to the Internet to pre-diagnose (often misdiagnose) their problems before even making an appointment.

Consequently, a clear, comprehensible explanation of what is the problem and what is the solution to the problem is crucial. If it is necessary to use technical terms, be sure to explain/define those terms for the patient. And provide visual aids to enhance and reinforce your explanation. The visual channel is central to the way we listen. Listening research suggests that we visualize as we listen, so *a good communicator takes us there visually*. The use of video images, for example, of the patient's mouth or teeth can be compelling and comprehensible for your patient.

Your *nonverbal* (vocal and visual) message is just as important as what you say verbally. Some research even suggests that the nonverbal is more important; as much as 93% of the impact of a message on a listener may be communicated through the vocal and visual channels.[9,10] So try to position yourself so you have eye contact with your patient as you conduct your consultation. This visual connection reassures your patient that you are a caring clinician, and eye contact enables you to process how your patient is responding to your diagnosis. Likewise, be sensitive to your care-giving demeanor. Communicate in a warm, expressive vocal tone and with pleasant facial expression. It may seem self-evident to communicate that you care, yet be aware that it is tempting to look at the radiographs or at your computer screen while conducting this interview. I can think of some of my own health care providers who never look at me during a diagnosis, being focused on their computer, even to the point of having their back to me!

The clinician–patient interaction does not stop with the initial interview. The patient is often present for treatment purposes. It also is important to maintain a clear, compassionate communication approach throughout any treatment process. This can be difficult, of course, because you are concentrating on the technical dimensions of the actual treatment. But it is important to patients that they know about and understand what it is that you are going to do and, then, what it is you are doing.

Then there is the post-treatment interaction in which you need to provide the patient with an explanation of what are the next steps in their dental care. You may want to use the teach-back method where you clarify with your patient that they understand what to do when they leave your office (i.e. *"Do not chew on this side for the rest of the day."*). After you explain the next steps, ask your patient to paraphrase back what it is they are going to do to be sure that they understand, and can do, what must be done to further their care.

Research has shown that the level of recall by a patient of post-operative instructions is low. It is helpful, therefore, to provide this guidance both orally and in a note or take-away instruction sheet that the patient can refer to later. While it is common practice to provide information for post-procedure immediate care, patients frequently also may need long-term guidance as to how long something may take to heal or respond to treatment, how the follow-up care might derail and how best to respond to any complications. Spending a few minutes with a patient at the end of the appointment exchanging pleasantries can also have a very positive effect on building trust and improving clinician–patient relationships.

Effective communication extends also to all care providers in your office. All play an important role in communicating with your patients. Just as you need to be an effective listener and an effective speaker in your interactions with patients, so too must your staff be responsible for ensuring that each patient has a positive communication experience – and everyone should make certain that the patient leaves with a clear understanding of *what is next* in terms of referrals, additional appointments and follow-up care.

Of course, the clinician–patient communication partnership brings with it *patient responsibilities*. While much of the work in health communication centers on the health care provider, patients need to be effective communicators as well. When a patient is in pain and anxious about what treatment must be undertaken, it can be a challenge to listen fully to the diagnosis and the treatment plan. And then the patient may often have to make a quick decision to go ahead with the treatment. This requires that they provide a full explanation of what is wrong, where the pain is and how painful it is. As they engage with the clinician, it is important to seek clarification through questions and paraphrases that allow them to have a clear understanding of what must be done to resolve the problem. If the issue is complicated, they may find it useful to have someone with them to help them ask the questions and to be *a second listener*, so that they have a full understanding of the problem and the treatment plan to be undertaken.

Good communication is the cornerstone of every effective clinical practice. Establishing a Communicating Practice is a challenge. It requires:

- A commitment to and appreciation of effective communication as an essential component of professional clinical practice
- A consistent effort to listen carefully and empathetically to the patient's verbal and nonverbal messages
- Strategic use of questions to enable an accurate diagnosis and responsive treatment
- Clear verbal explanations at every step in the diagnosis, treatment and follow-up
- Engagement of the entire staff in good communication with patients and with each other
- Application of the clinical observation skills described throughout the chapters in this manual.

Barriers to establishing a Communicating Practice can be significant. If you are dealing with a person in pain, they are probably emotionally upset. The patient brings their own communication approach and abilities, which are often a further variable. A patient who has *chronic pain*, also may have seen many clinicians. As well as being apprehensive, they may be angry and critical of past practitioners. Many may be confused, initially having difficulty in explaining their problem and frustrated by many diagnoses. Some may be more interested in describing who they have seen and what their past diagnoses have been. Some might appear evasive, omitting key parts of their history. Some probably are already convinced of a diagnosis and unreceptive to questioning and advice. In addition, you are dealing with your own staff who bring their own issues to the workplace. Furthermore, there are often time pressures. No matter how much you may want to empathetically listen to your patient, you also may have other patients waiting for you too. Additionally, *language differences* might require an interpreter. This can change the communication dynamics as you are then dealing with another individual and their interpretative nuances of what you are communicating and what the patient may be trying to communicate with you.

Clearly, effective communication in a clinical setting is not something that just happens, and it is not something that should be assumed. It takes time and commitment to create and to maintain a Communicating Practice. And it requires a significant level of *communication competency*[2] in which the communicators understand what they are doing, why they are doing it, and to care about it, while at the same time functioning with a high professional degree of clinical competency. The results, however, will be satisfying to you, your staff and your patients.

Chapter 3

Causes of Pain in the Orofacial Region

Vishal R. Aggarwal, Alex J. Moule and M. Lamar Hicks

Introduction

Pain is *"an unpleasant sensory and emotional experience associated with actual or potential tissue damage or described in terms of such damage"*.[11] It is a multidimensional experience encompassing somatic sensations and unpleasant emotions that can disrupt every aspect of a person's life and cause suffering and psychological distress. A patient's perception of pain and their reaction to it are influenced by these factors. All pain is real, but unfortunately from a diagnostic perspective, it is only the patient who feels the pain. Pain is invisible to the clinician.

Emotional factors aside, a patient's physical experience of pain is governed by certain neurophysiological mechanisms. The pain experienced can be described symptomatically, but can also be explained or defined biologically. The primary emphasis in this manual is on the former, that is, how patients describe pain and how descriptors and descriptions help to establish a diagnosis.

In any discussion of orofacial pain, certain terms need to be defined:

- *Threshold* refers to the initial level at which pain is experienced and differs from individual to individual due to underlying genetic, physiologic, social and environmental factors.
- *Adaptation* is the state in which an individual no longer feels pain over time or feels limited pain to a "normally" painful stimulus. The pain response is diminished over time.
- *Localization* refers to a specific site of pain that can easily be identified within an organ or tissue.
- *Hyperalgesia* is an increased response to a painful stimulus.
- *Hypoalgesia* is a reduced pain response to a stimulus that is normally more painful. This altered pain state may be the result of adaptation.

- *Allodynia* is a painful response to a normally innocuous or non-painful stimulus.
- *Neuralgia* is an intense burning or stabbing pain, usually intermittent or paroxysmal, that follows the course or distribution of a nerve.
- *Neurogenic pain* refers to pain that arises or originates in a nerve or in nervous tissue.
- *Neuropathic* refers to chronic pain resulting from injury to the peripheral or central nervous system.

Orofacial pain is generally defined as pain originating below the orbitomeatal line, above the neck and anterior to the ears.[12] A broader definition is used in sections of this manual.

Orofacial pain may be acute or chronic. Acute pain often occurs as a result of trauma, injury or a disease such as cancer or infection. Acute pain that resolves with treatment may still progress to chronic pain. This type of pain, which accompanies neurogenic inflammation, can present confusing symptoms and can only be diagnosed with proper attention to the patient's history. While acute pain is transient and protective, chronic pain can persist for months or years and is generally non-protective. Some chronic pain conditions appear to have no organic cause and their etiology is poorly understood.

The orofacial region has a very complex anatomy in contrast to many other regions of the body. It is also exposed to a wide variety of external influences. Thus, many pain conditions are possible. In addition, the region is innervated by several major somatic nerve trunks: the trigeminal, facial, glossopharyngeal and vagus cranial nerves, and the first, second and third cervical spinal nerves. This major regional neural complex allows referral of pain not only within the orofacial region, but also from other regions of the body. Due to this, the classification of orofacial pain conditions is difficult, especially those conditions

Diagnosing Dental and Orofacial Pain: A Clinical Manual, First Edition. Edited by Alex J. Moule and M. Lamar Hicks.
© 2017 John Wiley & Sons, Ltd. Published 2017 by John Wiley & Sons, Ltd.
Companion website: www.wiley.com/go/moule/dental_and_orofacial_pain

that are chronic, are of unknown etiology and are influenced by psychosocial factors.

A general classification[13] of head, neck and face conditions associated with orofacial pain includes:

- Intraoral pain conditions
- Musculoskeletal pain conditions affecting the jaw (temporomandibular disorders)
- Medical conditions that directly cause pain in or refer pain to the orofacial region.

Causes of orofacial pain

Dental causes

While there is a confusing array of causes of orofacial pain, by far the greatest number are of dental origin.[14] Dental pain can vary in severity from mild sensitivity or tenderness to severe diffuse debilitating pain. Pain can emanate from the dentin (dentin sensitivity), from inflammation of the dental pulp or from the periodontal supporting tissues. The quality of pain varies widely, but dentally related orofacial pain commonly starts as a sharp stabbing pain that progressively becomes dull and throbbing. The pain can be provoked or spontaneous. Sharp pain of momentary duration may be due to fluid movement in the dentinal tubules.[15] This commonly occurs when dentin is exposed by gingival recession, abrasion or dentinal erosion, or by dentinal cracks or fractures. Deep throbbing pain usually involves the pulp and the periapical tissues.

After a thorough clinical and radiographic examination, acute dental pain is relatively easy to diagnose. Common initiating factors are thermal changes and biting forces. Dental pain can also be referred to a distant site in the same jaw or the opposing jaw, making diagnosis more difficult. It rarely crosses the midline, and then only if the cause is in or around the midline. Pain from the soft and hard supporting tissues of the teeth is usually due to acute periodontitis, ulceration or food impaction. Unlike pulpal pain, which varies in intensity and may be difficult to localize, soft tissue pain is usually constant and easy to localize.

Mucosal causes

Many local and general conditions can cause mucosal erosions or ulcerations, which can lead to localized intraoral pain.[16–19] Erosions are superficial breaches in the epithelium which appear reddish in color and may be covered by a yellowish exudate. Ulcerations are breaches in the epithelium involving the underlying lamina propria. It is important to differentiate between an ulcer and tooth-related pathology. Ulcers are open sores, generally yellowish or grayish in color, surrounded by an erythematous margin. Ulcers and erosions are sensitive to touch and aggravated by acidic, salty or spicy foods. They are usually easily diagnosed. Most patients are aware that an ulcer is present, but anecdotally patients may complain of toothache when the main cause of their discomfort is an ulcer.

The most painful lesions are aphthous ulcers, herpes-related ulcerations, erythema multiforme (a Type IV hypersensitivity) and blistering conditions including pemphigus and pemphigoid.

Pain from temporomandibular disorder (TMD)

Temporomandibular disorder (TMD) is a general term reflecting dysfunction of the masticatory system. Pain from TMD typically originates in the masticatory muscles, in the temporomandibular joint (TMJ) or from chronic neuropathic mechanisms in response to this.[20]

TMD can present as:

- Masticatory muscle disorders (muscle pain)
- Arthralgia (temporomandibular joint pain)
- Headache associated with TMD (headache).

Masticatory muscle disorders (muscle pain)

The most common cause of non-odontogenic orofacial pain is masticatory muscle pain.[20] The act of chewing involves the simultaneous bilateral movement of the elevator muscles of the jaw, principally the temporalis, masseter and pterygoid muscles (Fig. 3-1).

Any inflammation, overuse or dysfunction of these muscles can result in the development of muscle pain. Patients often unknowingly contract their jaw muscles during periods of stress. This can result in muscle pain. The pain may be acute when there is significant damage or inflammation (e.g. in trismus) or dull, which is characteristic of chronic muscle dysfunction. Pain from the muscles of mastication can be referred to teeth or to other sites in the orofacial region.[21]

The depressor muscles of the mandible, which include the lateral pterygoid, digastric, mylohyoid and geniohyoid, can also become inflamed and painful (Fig. 3-2).

Temporomandibular joint pain

The mandible is articulated with the temporal bone by a bilateral hinged joint, the temporomandibular joint (TMJ). An articular disc is positioned between the head of the condyle and the articular eminence of the temporal bone, separating the joint into two halves. This arrangement allows the condyle to first rotate and then with increased jaw opening to slide (translate) forward. The anterior portion of the disc is attached to the superior head of the lateral pterygoid muscle (Fig. 3-3).

(A)

(B)

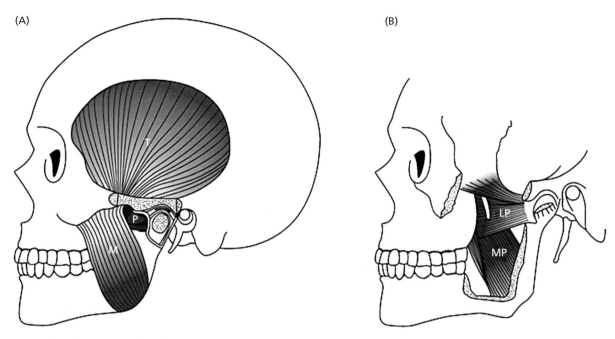

Fig. 3-1 (A) The major muscles of mastication: masseter (M), temporalis (T) and pterygoid (P). (B) The lateral (LP) and medial (MP) pterygoid muscles.

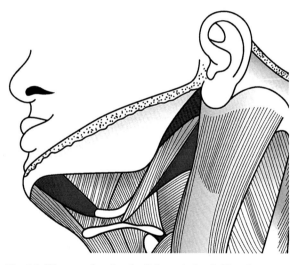

Fig. 3-2 Diagram showing (red) the anterior (left) and posterior (right) bellies of the digastric muscle which depress the mandible.

The term arthralgia refers to pain caused by inflammation within the joint capsule.[20] It is characterized by tenderness to palpation of the lateral pole of the condyle or pain in the joint with wide opening. Pain may be accompanied by joint noises and restriction of movement. The pain is usually felt in front of the ear and can involve muscle dysfunction, degenerative joint disease and disc derangements. Condylar pathoses are rarely involved.

Headaches associated with TMD

Headaches may be experienced secondary to temporomandibular disorders.[22] These are usually bilateral with a dull character. Palpation of a trigger point in the affected musculature, usually the temporalis, will initiate or exacerbate the headache.

Referral of pain from neck

Pain can be referred into the orofacial region when the cervical spine (Fig. 3-4) is affected by injury or disc disorders. Contributing factors are weakened musculature or poor posture.[23] The co-existence of TMD and cervicogenic problems is well documented. Pain referral from the structures of the cervical spine and associated nerves and musculature can contribute to orofacial pain, particularly chronic orofacial pain conditions.

Cervicogenic pain is usually unilateral and felt in the occipital or temporal regions and in other orofacial structures. Limitation of movement and the initiation of any symptoms during rotational and then vertical movements involving flexion and extension of the neck are strongly suggestive of cervicogenic pain. Severe pain (withdrawal) when the upper cervical spine is palpated is also indicative of cervicogenic pain. Palpation of trigger points in the posterior cervical muscles, which include the splenius, levator scapulae, longissimus and trapezius, may "set off" a frontal headache.[24]

Paranasal sinus-related orofacial pain

Four pairs of air-filled paranasal sinuses are located in the skull on either side of the nose (Fig. 3-5). These help reduce the weight of the skull, improve voice resonance and moisturize the nasal cavity. Inflammation of the nasal cavity and these paranasal sinuses, termed rhinosinusitis, can result in a variety of orofacial pain conditions.

The largest paranasal sinus is the maxillary sinus, which connects with the middle meatus of the nasal cavity through the ostium. Diseases involving the maxillary sinus often cause orofacial pain.[25] Maxillary sinus pain can range from severe pain and congestion

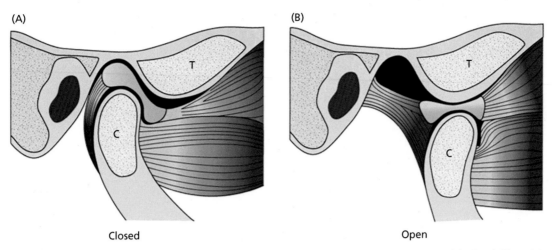

Fig. 3-3 Diagram of a section through the temporomandibular joint. In closed position (A) with the condylar head (C) positioned in the glenoid fossa with the articular disc (green) situated above and anterior to it. In open position (B) where the condylar head and the disc (green) have moved forward and are positioned over the temporal bone (T).

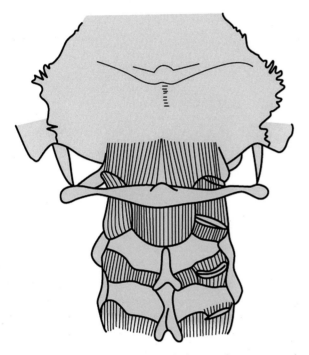

Fig. 3-4 Diagram of back of the neck showing the structures of the cervical spine and occipital bone (yellow). Damage to the cervical vertebrae or the discs can cause localized pain and referral to the orofacial region.

in the local area with or without associated systemic conditions to a constant mid-face headache. Pain may be aggravated by postural changes. It can also involve dental symptoms including thermal sensitivity in maxillary molar teeth, infra-orbital tenderness and pain on postural or atmospheric changes. Inflammation of the mucosa around the highly sensitive ostium contributes significantly to the pain experienced during an acute episode of sinusitis.

Odontogenic infection can spread into the maxillary sinus producing a sinusitis. Unilateral, chronic recalcitrant rhinosinusitis, an inflammatory process that involves the paranasal sinuses and persists for 12 weeks or longer, is strongly suggestive of an odontogenic origin.[26]

Trigeminal nerve pain

The trigeminal nerve (CN V) is the largest cranial nerve.[27] It supplies sensory innervation to the face, mouth, ocular structures and scalp. Its mandibular division supplies motor fibers to the major muscles of mastication, the anterior belly of the digastric, the tensor veli palatini and the tensor tympani. The nerve originates in the trigeminal nerve root or ganglion in the brainstem and then branches into three divisions: mandibular, maxillary and ophthalmic (Fig. 3-6).

The nerve can be involved in many orofacial pain conditions. An aberration in the trigeminal nerve can lead to trigeminal neuralgia (TN), a very severe pain condition. TN is the most common neurological cause of orofacial pain. It presents as an electric shock-like pain that lasts for a few seconds to minutes in the region innervated by the trigeminal nerve. It is usually unilateral. The pain is excruciating and can be triggered by an ipsilateral trigger point activated by touch, talking, chewing, swallowing or surface temperature change. TN commonly results from compression of the nerve by a lesion or a blood vessel as a consequence of the aging process. If it occurs in younger patients, multiple sclerosis should be suspected. A space-occupying lesion in the brain can also compress the nerve and result in TN. Trauma to the trigeminal nerve can lead to persistent pain and numbness.

Facial nerve-related orofacial pain

The facial nerve (CN VII) has sensory, autonomic (preganglionic parasympathetic) and motor functions.[27] Its primary function involves motor control of the muscles of facial expression and the smallest muscle in the body, the stapedius muscle in the middle ear (Fig. 3-7).

It is also responsible via its intracranial chorda tympani branch for taste sensation on the anterior two-thirds of the tongue. Its five extracranial branches pass through the parotid gland, but do not innervate it. The facial nerve does provide parasympathetic

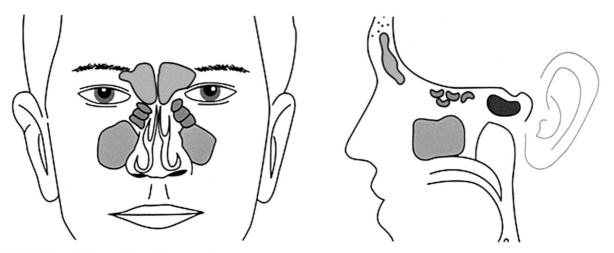

Fig. 3-5 The relative position of the paranasal sinuses: maxillary (yellow), frontal (purple), ethmoid (blue) and sphenoid (red).

(A)   (B)

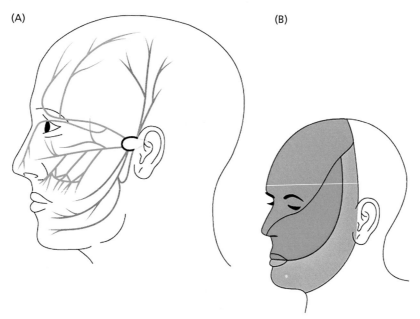

Fig. 3-6 Representation of the trigeminal nerve (CN V), the largest of the cranial nerves. (A) The course of the nerve and (B) the areas of sensory innervation of the three divisions: mandibular (ochre), maxillary (green) and ophthalmic (blue). Adapted from: https://www.google.com.kw/search?q=trigeminal+nerve&biw=1325&bih=794&source=lnms&tbm=isch&sa=X&sqi=2&ved=0CAYQ_AUoAWoVChMI-p-Lo-iYxwIVCMUUCh0IfgfD#imgrc=yMVAsT16OBSMGM%3A (accessed 8 August, 2015).

(A)   (B)

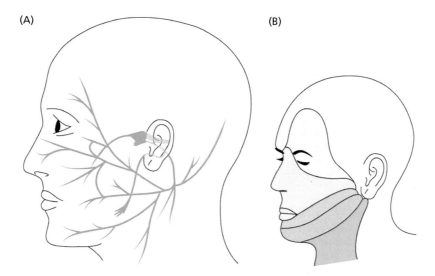

Fig. 3-7 The facial nerve (A) showing the course of the nerve and (B) the sensory innervation of its five divisions: temporal (ochre), buccal (purple), zygomatic (blue), mandibular (orange) and cervical (green). Adapted from: https://www.google.com.kw/search?q=facial+nerve&biw=1325&bih=794&source=lnms&tbm=isch&sa=X&sqi=2&ved=0CAYQ_AUoAWoVChMIsMeC2eiYxwIVh-0UCh3osgxX#imgrc=5SRImR3VhvA3mM%3A (accessed 8 August 2015).

fibers through its chorda tympani branch to the sub-mandibular, sublingual and lacrymal glands. CN VII also provides sensory innervation to the earlobe.

Orofacial pain originating from the facial nerve is rare as its sensory function is secondary to its motor functions. Pain can occur when the varicella zoster virus reactivates in the geniculate (facial nerve) ganglion producing the well-known signs and symptoms of Ramsay Hunt syndrome, an acute peripheral facial neuropathy with erythematous vesicular rash of the skin of the ear canal, auricle (herpes zoster oticus) and mucous membrane of the oropharynx. It also can cause facial paralysis and hearing loss. The main differences between Ramsay Hunt syndrome and other facial shingles outbreaks are the facial paralysis and the distribution of the vesicles along a branch of the facial nerve.

Glossopharyngeal nerve-related orofacial pain

The glossopharyngeal nerve (CN IX) is a mixed nerve.[27] Among its many functions, it receives sensory impulses from the pharynx, the middle ear and the posterior one-third of the tongue. It also receives special sensory impulses of taste from the posterior one-third of the tongue. Parasympathetic fibers supply the parotid gland and motor fibers supply the stylopharyngeus muscle (Fig. 3-8).

An aberration in the glossopharyngeal nerve can lead to glossopharyngeal neuralgia, a rare and debilitating condition that causes severe pain in the throat, tonsils, tongue and middle ear. The pain is caused by compression of the glossopharyngeal nerve by blood vessels that run in close proximity to the nerve. Characteristically the pain is sharp and stabbing and lasts for a few minutes. It is brought on by swallowing, coughing, talking or laughing.

Occipital nerve pain

The occipital nerves are two pairs of spinal nerves (greater and lesser occipital) that originate between the second and third vertebra and innervate the posterior area of the scalp.[27]

Occipital neuralgia, an extremely severe and debilitating painful condition with frequent paroxysms, may occur after trauma to the nerve(s), entrapment of the nerves under the trapezius or capitis muscles, or spondylosis of the upper cervical spine (C1–C2). The pain is usually unilateral and felt in the neck and back of the head. At times it can mimic migraine, eye pain or even dental pain.[28] The nerve may be tender and the pain is relieved by administration of a local anesthetic.

Superior laryngeal nerve

The superior laryngeal nerve is a branch of the vagus nerve (CN X) (Fig. 3-9). It is responsible for motor innervation to the cricothyroid muscle, which allows changes in voice pitch.[27]

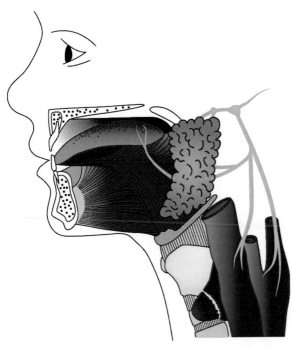

Fig. 3-8 Diagram of the course (orange) of the glossopharyngeal nerve. The nerve supplies sensory fibers to the pharynx, middle ear and posterior one-third of the tongue (including taste). Adapted from: https://www.google.com.kw/search?q=glossopharyngeal+nerve&biw=1325&bih=794&source=lnms&tbm=isch&sa=X&sqi=2&ved=0CAYQ_AUoAWoVCh MIypqKtemYxwIVw1oUCh1t3wGu#imgrc=RN5bvb0 veX_aMM%3A (accessed 8 August 2015).

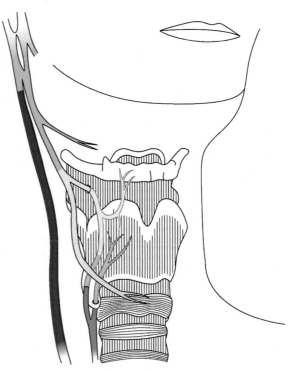

Fig. 3-9 Course (yellow) of the superior laryngeal nerve, a branch of the vagus nerve (CN X). The nerve innervates the cricothyroid muscle. Adapted from: https://www.google.com.kw/search?q=superior+laryngeal+nerve&biw=1325&bih=794&source=lnms&tbm=isch&sa=X&ved=0CAYQ_AUoAWoVCh MIkO6xyOqYxwIVhbUUCh2eDQ1I#imgrc=W7t_ Hu6om6ZQqM%3A (accessed 8 August 2015).

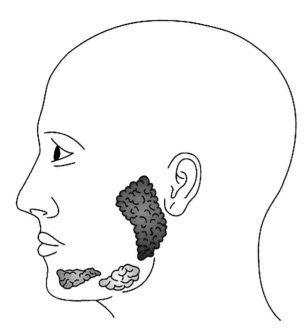

Fig. 3-10 Sagittal view of the face showing the relative position of the major salivary glands: parotid (orange), submandibular (green) and sublingual (blue). The parotid gland is situated superficially in front of the ear on the side of the face. The other glands are situated sublingually medial to the inner surface of the horizontal ramus of the mandible. Adapted from http://www.zadehmd.com/images/salivaryNew.jpg (accessed 8 August 2015).

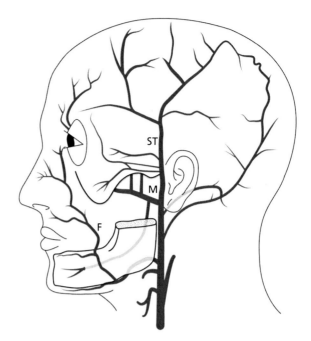

Fig. 3-11 Blood supply to the face with main branches highlighted: maxillary (M), facial (F) and superficial temporal (ST).

Paralysis of this nerve results in hoarseness. Superior laryngeal neuralgia is caused by compression or damage to this nerve. It presents as an electric shock-like pain on one side of the throat just below the mandible and ear. The pain can be triggered by swallowing, shouting or turning the head to one side. A patient may be unable to speak without pain.

Salivary gland pain

There are three pairs of major salivary glands, two pairs in the mandible and one in front of each ear (Fig. 3-10). Hundreds of minor salivary glands are also located throughout the oral cavity within the submucosa of the oral mucosa.[29] Saliva from each of the major glands is secreted into the oral cavity through ducts that connect the gland to the oral cavity. The parotid duct opens adjacent to the upper molar teeth, the submandibular and sublingual glands anteriorly below the tongue.

Salivary gland-related pain[30] can arise through blockage of the duct, usually by a salivary stone or calculus. The pain often becomes intense just before eating when increased salivary output causes pressure and swelling in the gland. Another cause is a benign or malignant tumor of a gland (e.g. pleomorphic adenomas or adenoid cystic carcinomas, respectively). A salivary gland can also become painful and swollen when a bacterial infection (acute bacterial sialadenitis) occurs. Viruses, including the mumps virus, can cause pain and bilateral swelling in salivary glands (usually the parotids). These infections are accompanied by systemic symptoms including fever, headaches, muscle aches, tiredness and loss of appetite.

Neurovascular causes of orofacial pain

Most of the blood supply to the head and neck is supplied by the carotid and vertebral arteries, with the external carotid artery supplying the areas of the head and neck external to the cranium (Fig. 3-11). The artery gives off six branches with the major branches being the maxillary, the facial and the superficial temporal arteries. The maxillary artery supplies the deeper structures of the face, while the facial and superficial temporal arteries generally supply superficial areas of the face.

Neurovascular pains are primarily viewed as arising from neuronal firing of nociceptors associated with intracranial blood vessels and dura. Pain can result from vascular disorders thought to involve constriction or dilatation of blood vessels. Until recently, migraine headaches were thought to be vascular in origin.

Cluster headaches are primary, unilateral headaches.[31] They are characterized by excruciating pain in the region of the trigeminal nerve (usually orbital or peri-orbital pain). They are usually accompanied by cranial autonomic signs including conjunctival injection, lacrimation, rhinorrhea and Horner's syndrome (unilateral ptosis and miosis). Pain tends to occur in clusters of one or two episodes of pain a day for weeks to months.

Giant cell arteritis[32] is the most common form of vasculitis in adults (almost all over the age of 50) and results in headaches, scalp tenderness, facial pain, joint pain, throat or tongue pain, and vision difficulties, including permanent loss of vision in one or both eyes.

The condition can be accompanied by one or more systemic manifestations including fever, cough, jaw claudication, arm pain during exercise, weight loss, depression, tiredness, night sweats or anorexia. Early diagnosis is critical, as delay in treatment can lead to vascular infarct and permanent blindness.

Cranial artery dissection[33,34] results from a tear in the inner layer of a cranial artery causing an intra-arterial hematoma. Subsequent extension can lead to occlusion of the artery, embolism, ischemia or compression of neural structures. Cranial artery dissection can occur spontaneously, from trauma or due to an existing arterial disease. The internal carotid artery is the most common vessel involved. Patients may present with headache and orofacial or cervical pain, which are usually severe and of sudden onset. The pain often involves the neck, jaw, face, ear, or periorbital or frontal-temporal regions. Horner's syndrome is a prominent feature.

Others causes of headache include neurovascular and vascular disorders (e.g. cluster headache), neuralgias (e.g. trigeminal neuralgia), intracranial infections (e.g. meningitis), intracranial lesions (e.g. tumors) and medication/substance withdrawal. Vasoconstriction caused by excessive smoking or caffeine consumption may be followed by a rebound dilatation, causing a *dull headache*. Prolonged or intense exercise, particularly at high altitude, can precipitate a headache.

Viral causes of orofacial pain

Certain viral infections can contribute to the development of orofacial pain. The most common of these are the herpes simplex viruses (HSV1 and 2). HSV1 is usually associated with oral infections.[35] These oral infections are characterized by blisters or balloon-like vesicles accompanied by fever, malaise, regional lymphadenopathy and difficulty in eating (dysphagia). They resolve in about two weeks. The virus then moves to a sensory nerve ganglion where it remains as a persistent latent virus until reactivated (cold sore).[36] A similar pattern of infection and reactivation occurs with the varicella zoster virus (VZV) (chicken pox virus). Reactivation of the virus can result in a painful varicella zoster infection (shingles) characterized by vesicles, which in the orofacial region commonly occurs in one of the three divisions of the trigeminal nerve. When the facial nerve is involved, vesicles appear and unilateral facial paralysis occurs (Ramsay Hunt syndrome). VZV infections can be accompanied or followed by severe neuralgia. Post-herpetic neuralgias can cause a continuous searing or burning pain that can continue for many weeks, months or even years.[37]

Neuropathic pain

Neuropathic pain involves the expression of pain-producing neuropeptides, including substance P and other neurokinins.[38] These neuropeptides are resistant to enzymatic breakdown, causing chronic neuropathic pain. Neuropathic pain requires treatment frequently involving anti-neuropathic drugs, which act on the central cholinergic system.[39]

The onset of neuropathic orofacial pain often coincides with a stressful life event that occurred just prior to the onset of pain. Behavioral extremes and psychological characteristics such as catastrophization, unrealistic expectations, aggression, drug and alcohol abuse, psychiatric conditions and depression can perpetuate the orofacial neuropathic pain condition.

Central sensitization

A constant barrage of nociceptive input from peripheral activity can lead to functional changes in the central nervous system.[40] Nociceptive neurons become hyper-excited to the extent that stimuli such as pressure and touch, which are normally innocuous, are perceived as painful. This phenomenon is known as central sensitization and can lead to persistent pain.

Central sensitization is typically observed in chronic pain disorders. In the orofacial region it can present as chronic temporomandibular pain or persistent idiopathic orofacial pain. Patients with these conditions may have concurrent chronic pain conditions such as fibromyalgia with its core symptom of chronic widespread pain or the associated disorder, irritable bowel syndrome.[41]

Heterotrophic pain

The complex anatomy of the neural structures of the orofacial region can result in referral of pain out of the region.[40] Pain from other sites or structures from outside the orofacial region can be referred into the region. This referred pain is termed *heterotrophic pain*.[42] Dental pain can be referred to another tooth, to a more remote site in the same jaw or to an opposing arch, but only on the same side. Pain referral from a dental cause does not cross the midline unless the source of the problem is in the midline. When this referred pain occurs, diagnosis can be more difficult and confusing for both the clinician and the patient, because the site to which the pain has been referred is not the source of the pain.

Intracranial lesions

Intracranial inflammation and neoplastic processes can result in pain in the orofacial region. The type of pain is dependent upon the anatomic location and the size of the lesion. An intra-cranial lesion should be considered if a patient presents with an initially (first off) severe headache of increasing severity or where orofacial pain is accompanied by systemic symptoms such as nausea and vomiting, visual disturbances or pupillary asymmetry, seizures or collapse, paresthesia or muscle dysfunction.[43]

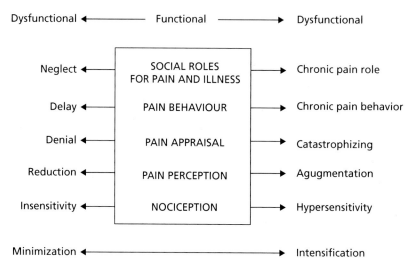

Fig. 3-12 Biopsychosocial model for chronic pain.[44,45]

Psychological aspects of pain experience

Pain experience is multifactorial (Fig. 3-12) and is modulated not just by neurochemical mediators, but also by psychosocial factors that act to inhibit pain signals via the limbic system and descending modulation. Thus, any discussion of pain must also include a patient's reaction to it, which is shaped by both sensory (physiologic) and emotional (psychological) components. In an effort to categorize pain, clinicians have categorized it into two divisions termed Axis I and Axis II:

- Axis I relates to the physical signs and symptoms of disease, and has two foundations:
  1. the source of the pain, and
  2. the presence or absence of an associated structural abnormality.
- Axis II relates to the *psychosocial impact* of the condition.

Axis I and II definitions are, however, not mutually exclusive, as pain from both has sensory and emotional components. It is now generally accepted that pain is better described using a *biopsychosocial model* (Fig. 3-12), which takes into consideration the sensory and emotional components. This is in counter-distinction to a *biomedical model* in which pain is described only in relation to signs and symptoms. In the biopsychosocial model, psychological factors influence the appraisal and perception of pain, and social factors shape the behavioral response of patients around their perceptions of their pain.[44,45] Pain can be intensified or minimized at each level, resulting in the dysfunction of the individual.

Dysfunctional minimization of pain can include congenital pain insensitivity, excessive pain reduction, excessive stoicism, and delay in seeking treatment or neglect of a person affected by pain.

In contrast, *dysfunctional intensification* of pain may include hypersensitivity, pain augmentation, catastrophizing and behaviors related to chronic illness and chronic occupation of the sick role.

The inclusion of the *construct of time* to the biopsychosocial model recognizes that the development of pain conditions may differ across biological and psychological phases and that prior development of pain may contribute to the present pain experience and behavior. Thus, reviewing the natural history of a patient's pain (e.g. the order and timing of development, and the course and remission of chronic pain and dysfunction) can yield insights into causal mechanisms and assist in diagnosis. Variability in a patient's expression of chronic pain across time does mean that different factors will predominate during the evolution and development of a particular pain condition. During the acute phase, biological factors may predominate. However, over time, psychological and social factors over time begin to account for symptoms and disability. These factors need to be identified and managed as part of an overall treatment program. Depression and anxiety are often prevalent in patients with chronic pain. In addition, psychological distress can be a factor in the development and maintenance of chronic pain. Psychosocial modulation also underlies the onset of persistent neuropathic orofacial pain and explains why such pain coincides with stressful life events (e.g. a divorce) that occurred just prior to the onset of a patient's pain. These factors need to be identified and managed as part of an overall treatment program.

Genetic factors affecting pain diagnosis

Genetic factors can modulate the response of an individual to their pain experience via pain beliefs, expectations, the placebo effect and the impact of psychosocial mediators. This explains the variability of the chronic pain experience between individuals, despite being exposed to the same stimuli.

Medical conditions that can cause orofacial pain

There are a number of medical illnesses that are accompanied by orofacial pain. These include:

- Oral manifestations of AIDS, including neuropathic pain, periodontitis and Kaposi's sarcoma.
- Digestive disorders causing oral ulceration, including malabsorption, ulcerative colitis and Crohn's disease.
- Iron, B_{12} and folate deficiencies (anemia), causing oral ulceration.
- Carcinomas (late stage), causing facial pain; the most common and the most severe is squamous cell carcinoma.
- Viral infections (varicella zoster and herpes simplex), leading to ulceration and neuralgia.
- Local fungal infections (erythematous candidiasis), causing ulceration and sensitivity of soft tissues.

- Autoimmune diseases, including erythema multiforme and erosive lichen planus, causing painful ulcerations in the oral mucosa.
- Psychological disease states and psychiatric disorders, resulting in the development of the pain.

Summary

It should be apparent from the above that the many causes and subsequent effects of orofacial pain on the individual are exceedingly complex and dauntingly varied. It will only be through a thorough understanding of the intimate relationship among anatomical, physiological, psychological and sociological factors that practitioners can hope to develop sound strategies to recognize, evaluate and then synthesize effective approaches for managing patients in pain. To fail in this undertaking dooms countless patients to lives where pain and suffering threaten and then destroy their quality of life and well-being. The importance of knowledge of the underlying anatomical structures and the origin of painful conditions cannot be overestimated.

Chapter 4

Gathering Information for an Accurate Pain Diagnosis

Alex J. Moule and M. Lamar Hicks

Introduction

The recording of a pain history requires thorough and complete questioning of the patient and must include relevant questioning on the medical history, past illnesses, hospitalizations, allergies, a history of accidents, a relevant social history and a detailed pain history and profile.

When diagnosing pain, history taking is more important than testing procedures. It is the history that dictates the tests to be performed. History is obtained by asking appropriate questions. Diagnosis is based on questioning and observing the patient:

- Knowing the questions to ask (*What should I ask?*)
- Analyzing the answers received (*What does this answer mean? What else do I need to know?*)
- Applying this information to establish a diagnosis.

CAUTION: Do not jump to conclusions before gathering and assessing the full facts. Mistakes often occur if practitioners gather insufficient information before a diagnosis is made.

Practically, the initial task for a general dental practitioner is relatively straightforward when assessing a patient in pain. It is to establish whether the patient has a:

- treatable dental problem;
- treatable non-dental problem (e.g. sinusitis); or
- problem that requires referral to a dental or medical specialist.

Once this broad sorting has been carried out, more specific diagnosis and treatment planning can occur for each condition. To place the patient into one of these categories can be relatively easy, but to get to this stage is not always so easy. Patients in pain are likely to be stressed. They may be poor historians. They may not have been able to sleep and may be taking pain medications, which can mask symptoms

and make assessment difficult. In addition, there are numerous causes of orofacial pain, often with confusing presentations, which make diagnosis difficult.[46]

Patients with chronic pain can carry a lot of *emotional baggage*, which can cloud answers to questions. Conversely, practitioners can confound the problem by preventing patients from explaining their pain problems completely.[47] Indeed, studies show that most general practitioners will interrupt a patient within a few seconds of the start of a conversation.[48]

Historically, Dyche and Swiderski[49] recommended that a typical pain history should involve recording the onset, duration, progression, frequency, location, radiation, quality, intensity, alleviating factors, aggravating factors, daily patterns, environmental factors, physical factors, prior episodes, associated systemic symptoms and current medication. Subsequently, many other groupings of pain history questions have been suggested.[50] These comprehensive lists are important in complex diagnostic situations, but from a diagnostic point of view, clinicians can find it difficult to recall and analyze all of these sometimes confusing and seemingly unconnected questions. Practically, not all questions are relevant to all situations.

Screening questions

The philosophy of this manual is one of using *directed questioning* and a *diagnostic tree*. This is where clinicians commence with a series of vertical *general screening questions* and then branch out into *specific screening questions* once an answer, a descriptor, or a test result directs them away from general questioning. The importance of being a good listener cannot be over emphasized. Sometimes a single descriptor can suggest a line of questioning. Other times it may be necessary to be patient and listen for an extended period of time until a line of questioning becomes obvious and a probable diagnosis becomes apparent.

Diagnosing Dental and Orofacial Pain: A Clinical Manual, First Edition. Edited by Alex J. Moule and M. Lamar Hicks.
© 2017 John Wiley & Sons, Ltd. Published 2017 by John Wiley & Sons, Ltd.
Companion website: www.wiley.com/go/moule/dental_and_orofacial_pain

It is a premise of this manual that diagnosis of orofacial pain is difficult unless a clinician is aware of, and can use, the specific screening questions for most orofacial disease states (dental pain, cluster headache, trigeminal neuralgia, cranial arteritis etc.). Diagnosing orofacial pain is made easier if clinicians routinely use sorting or screening questions and utilize a 'diagnostic tree' (Fig. 4-1) to suggest further questioning and investigations. It is the responses to screening questions that direct the order and selection of the specific screening questions. It is the responses that help to confirm or deny a possible diagnosis and suggest useful testing methods.

Screening questions for an orofacial pain diagnosis have been grouped into seven broad groups (see below). Specific screening questions for each common orofacial pain condition and the relevance of each question will be found in each chapter. The manner in which screening questions are asked may vary from clinician to clinician according to personal preference and personality, but for orofacial pain, initial screening should include the following:

1. Basic information gathering	*How may I help you?*
	What do you think is the cause of your pain?
2. Pain description	*What sort of pain are you having?*
	Do you have pain to heat, cold or sweets?
3. The site of the pain	*Where is the pain?*
	Can you put your finger on where the pain is?
4. Time analysis	*When did the pain start?*
	Where did the pain start?
5. Factors influencing the pain	*Does anything make the pain worse?*
	Does anything make the pain better?
	Does medication help to relieve the pain?
6. Psychological and lifestyle factors	*Are you under stress or pressure?*
	Have you been able to sleep?
7. Associated general symptoms	*Does anything else happen when you are in pain?*

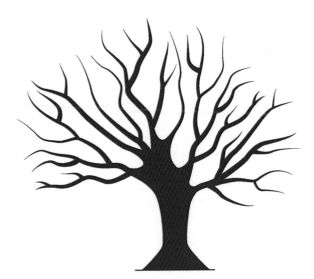

Fig. 4-1 Diagnosis of orofacial pain can be made easier if clinicians use directed *questioning* and a *diagnostic tree*, where responses to a series of *general screening questions*, a descriptor or a test result directs questioning towards *screening questions for specific disease states.*

Basic information gathering

What can I do for you (*How may I help you*)?

The first screening questions are designed for *basic information gathering* and establish the reason for the visit and the patient's understanding of their current pain problem. The questions should be phrased in a manner that puts the patient at ease and allows them to explain their problem. Questioning must be in plain language that a patient understands. Patients in pain need time to explain their problem. Remember, the initial problem discussed by the patient may not, in fact, be the main problem. Furthermore, the order in which a patient reports problems may not reflect their relative clinical importance.[47]

Special attention should be paid to responses to the general questions, *"What can I do for you?"* or *"How may I help you?"* Much can be gained by analyzing the patient's responses to these initial queries. These responses help to identify:

- the problem or chief complaint.
- a language problem the patient may have.

  NOTE: In some circumstances pain remains undiagnosed only because a patient has not been able to communicate the problem to the practitioner. This is a problem particularly with long-standing chronic pain. The practitioner should not judge the patient to be unintelligent just because they cannot communicate in a given language. If a language problem exists, an interpreter may be required.
- the emotional state of the patient, their level of anxiety, fear, distress or even anger towards current or past clinicians or treatment (Fig. 4-2). What the patient says and their body language may not be in accord. If a satisfactory diagnostic process is to be undertaken, emotions need to be recognized, acknowledged and addressed where possible.

  NOTE: Highly anxious patients expect and report more pain than they actually feel.[51]
- the expectations of the patient. (*"Can you help me? You have to help me! You will not be able to help me."*)
- the urgency of the patient's treatment needs. (Just discomfort or a severe pain that needs immediate attention.) (*"How bad is this pain?"* e.g. *"tolerable"* or *"I-can't-stand-this-anymore."*)
- whether the patient is involved in litigation. Pending litigation or ongoing insurance claims can influence both the patient's historical reporting and their interpretation of the pain. It also highlights the clinician's need for accuracy in recording every aspect of the pain history.
- the patient's response patterns. Different patients can exhibit dissimilar response patterns when describing pain, each of which has to be dealt with in a different way. Some of these patterns are described as *historical, diagnostic, factual* or *evasive.*

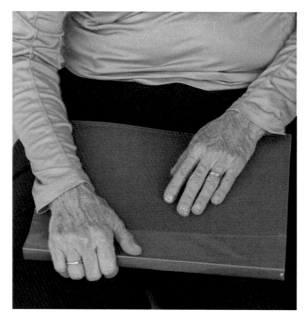

Fig. 4-2 Be wary of patients with chronic pain who give a long explanation of a problem, who are particularly critical of past treatment and other practitioners and who attend for consultation with dossiers containing a comprehensive array of past reports and records. Many need psychological assessment as well as any physical treatment.

Historical reporting

Historical reporting does little to assist with the identification of the patient's problems (*"I saw so-and-so and he/she said such and such…"*). While it is sometimes helpful to know who the patient has already consulted, and what tests may have been used, historical reporting often clouds the issue and does little to explain the patient's actual pain problem. It can also be extremely time wasting. Allowing a patient to discuss the opinions of other practitioners can also influence the diagnosis.

Be wary of patients who are openly critical of other practitioners, particularly patients who fit into an historical response pattern and bring with them a dossier of other practitioners' reports and opinions. This can negatively influence the diagnostic process. It may also be a red flag for a patient who is suffering from neuropathic facial pain where management has been and is unlikely to be successful.

Self-diagnosing patients

Similar to the historical patient, the *self-diagnostic* patient gives little information on their pain state, but rather their interpretation of it. (*"I thought my pain was such and such, but then I thought it was…"*). These patients need to be tactfully informed that first you need to know the actual symptoms they have experienced previously, or are experiencing now, before a diagnosis can be made.

Factual reporting

Patients who report their pain in a *factual* manner make diagnosis and treatment a lot easier. Factual patients give a clear and accurate description of the

pain, use descriptors that are easy to understand and provide an accurate timeline.

Evasive patients

Patients can evade answering specific questions for many reasons, some of which are valid. Nevertheless, unless there is an honest exchange between the patient and the practitioner, an accurate diagnosis is difficult to achieve. If a satisfactory and trusting rapport cannot be established, early referral of the patient is indicated.

When confronted with an evasive patient who does not report factually or gets off track into an unrelated topic, gently guide them back to the immediate problem. Explain that you need to know the full story about their problem rather than their personal or another person's interpretation of it.

Suggested Statement: *If I am going to help you with your pain problem, I need to know first about the pain you have experienced and exactly what you are feeling right now.*

RULES of THUMB:

- Never accept a diagnosis without confirming it yourself.
- Always assume the patient is identifying the wrong condition, the wrong area or the wrong tooth until you prove otherwise.
- Be aware that patients can compartmentalize their pain descriptions, telling you only what they think you need to know.

Further basic information gathering

What do you think is the cause of your pain?

There are times when a patient is well aware of the cause or where a cause-and-effect relationship exists between the pain and a past event. This information can be a valuable aid to diagnosis. It allows the patient to express in words their understanding of the cause. It also provides an insight into the patient's opinions or beliefs. Furthermore, asking the patient to discuss causation allows them to voice frustrations and inform the clinician about their perception of blame directed at past treatment and clinicians. However, asking patients for this information is not always helpful. Many patients are poor historians. As happens frequently, they may attribute the cause of their pain to a past treatment or associated event that is, in fact, unrelated. While a patient's belief on the cause of orofacial pain has to be respected, it is only with proper diagnosis that it can be confirmed.

In the chapters of this manual the importance of listening to a patient and asking the correct and appropriate questions is emphasized. In particular, answers to questioning are analyzed to draw attention to the meanings and importance of descriptors and descriptions.

Chapter 5

Analyzing Patients in Pain – Describing Pain and the Importance of Descriptors

Alex J. Moule and M. Lamar Hicks

What sort of pain are you having?

The question *"What sort of pain are you having?"* will elicit a variety of responses. Some patients can describe the pain accurately, whereas others have difficulty putting words to their experience. Pain descriptions are influenced not only by a particular pain, but also by the level of the arousal of the brain stem prior to the pain experience, the patient's emotional state, and *language idiosyncrasies* and ethnically determined behaviors. Pain descriptions are also affected by the intensity and type of pain being experienced. With recent advances in functional brain imaging, the complexity and plasticity of the brain, along with its anatomical and functional reorganization in the presence of chronic pain, are being subjected to more sophisticated and intensive investigation. There is a beginning recognition that central plasticity is an important feature of the chronic pain experience.[52]

> *A patient be subject to pain arising in different parts of the body simultaneously, the stronger blunts the other.*
> Hippocrates, 5th century BC

The question *"Do you have any reaction to heat or cold?"* is closely linked with *"What sort of pain are you having?"* and should be asked early on, as an affirmative answer almost always identifies the pain as being of dental origin and immediately prompts the clinician to move laterally along the diagnostic tree to screen for a dental cause. Rarely do other medical conditions have a trigger in the teeth, although maxillary sinusitis, trigeminal neuralgia or pre-trigeminal neuralgia may present in this way. The descriptors used by patients with these medical conditions are, however, usually different and distinctive. The diagnostic implications of thermal sensitivity are discussed elsewhere in this manual (see Chapter 7).

Severity

Patients will usually describe the type of pain they are experiencing and give an indication of the severity of the pain. Patients indicate severity both verbally and non-verbally. The information provided on severity should be recorded in the patient's words. Unfortunately there is no infallible way of measuring pain or feeling what a patient is feeling. A visual analogue scale (VAS), where a patient rates pain using a scale of 0 to 10, or other similar numerical scale is therefore helpful in assessing the patient's personal interpretation of the severity of what they are experiencing. In the VAS, the zero represents *no pain* and 10 is the *worst pain* the patient can imagine (Fig. 5-1). This helps the practitioner to determine the urgency of a treatment intervention. For chronic pain patients, baseline VAS assessment is also helpful to the clinician for assessing a patient's response to treatment over time. For example, it is not uncommon for chronic pain patients to report they are not getting any better, whereas reference to the VAS shows in fact that their pain experiences are diminishing in intensity or frequency.

Descriptors

When describing pain, it is necessary to be aware that patients will use *descriptors* that are often very specific for different pain states. Thus, when taking a pain history it is imperative to *record the exact words a patient uses in describing his or her pain*. Even if one of the many assessment forms that are available for recording pain histories is used, exact descriptors should be recorded at the time of examination. Although the descriptors used and the manner in which the patient describes the severity of the pain

Diagnosing Dental and Orofacial Pain: A Clinical Manual, First Edition. Edited by Alex J. Moule and M. Lamar Hicks.
© 2017 John Wiley & Sons, Ltd. Published 2017 by John Wiley & Sons, Ltd.
Companion website: www.wiley.com/go/moule/dental_and_orofacial_pain

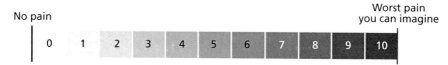

Fig. 5-1 The use of a simple visual analogue scale allows a patient to describe the intensity of their personal present and past pain experiences. It is a useful means of recording the current pain intensity, as well as changes in intensity that occur over time with treatment.

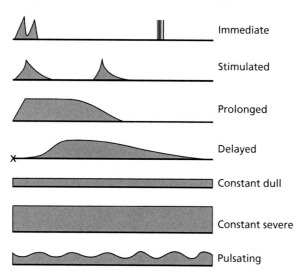

Fig. 5-2 Representation of patterns of a patient's pain experience. Pattern and intensity recorded in relation to a linear time line. The height of the line indicates intensity, and the shape of the line indicates the pattern of the pain experienced.

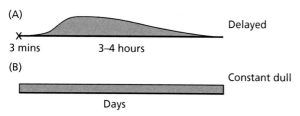

Figs 5-3 A and B. Representation of patterns of a patient's pain experience. Time detail can be entered in more detail below a diagram. If stimulated, the point of stimulation (x) is marked as the start point. In the first diagram (A), pain experience is delayed for some minutes after stimulation but then builds in intensity and lasts for hours before slow dissipation. In the second diagram (B), the patient described constant dull pain that has lasted for days.

may seem unimportant at the time, this information often proves invaluable when reviewing a diagnosis and recording changes in the pain profile over time. As well as recording pain descriptors, it is helpful when taking a pain history to also draw a representation of the type of pain the patient is reporting using a line diagram (Fig. 5-2). Adding the construct of time under the diagram completes the diagrammatic representation (Fig. 5-3).

This type of recording is particularly helpful in complex diagnostic situations, especially for ease of recall when a patient returns after an absence. In addition to recording the word descriptions the patient uses, line drawings can be used to characterize the type and severity of the pain. Constant mild pain,

constant severe pain, stimulated pain, prolonged stimulated pain, pulsating pain and pains that have a daily pattern (clusters) or random initiation (trigeminal neuralgia) can all be illustrated diagrammatically. These diagrams can be referred to later when confirming a diagnosis.

Similarly many other pain conditions follow patterns that can be represented diagrammatically (Figs 5-4 and 5-5).

From a practical point of view, it is much easier to recall a diagram when reviewing a patient's file than trying to read through a set of written notes. A pain diary can be useful when assessing patients with chronic pain. Any changes in pain throughout the day, such as its intensity, triggers or patterns, can be recorded (*see web appendix*). This is especially important when assessing the effect of medication. For most patients it is important that the diary only be kept for short periods of time and, if possible, placed in the patient's records, so that they do not rely on it to remind them they are in pain.

Importance of descriptors in diagnosis of orofacial pain

Patients usually describe pain using *sensory descriptors* (*the type of pain*). However, descriptors can also be *affective* (*what it is doing*) or *evaluative* (*about the pain*). Patients can also use diagnostic terms for pain (*what they think it is*). There are useful questionnaires that describe the importance of descriptors. The *McGill Pain Questionnaire* for example was designed to provide a quantitative measure of clinical pain that could be analyzed statistically.[54,55] It lists over 70 descriptive words, divided into 20 different categories that patients can use to describe pain. It applies a numerical value to each pain descriptor, thus allowing the progress of a patient to be monitored over time.

Not all patients can describe their symptoms eloquently, but the words (*descriptors*) a patient uses are very significant and often suggest a diagnosis and/or a line of questioning. It is important not only to hear the words, but also to interpret the meaning of these descriptors. When a patient has difficulty describing pain, take care not to suggest specific descriptors; instead, ask the patient to use any and as many words they feel are appropriate.

Some descriptors are specifically related to specific pain states, while others are informative for the type of pain and its effect on the patient. Not all of these

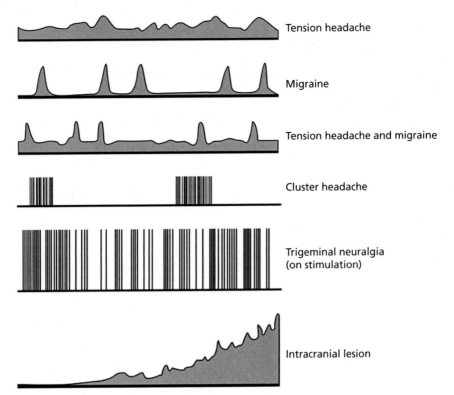

Tension headache

Migraine

Tension headache and migraine

Cluster headache

Trigeminal neuralgia (on stimulation)

Intracranial lesion

Fig. 5-4 Representation of patterns of a patient's pain experience. Pain patterns can be specific for a specific pain condition (adapted from Lance, J.W. *Mechanism and Management of Headache*, 5th ed).[53]

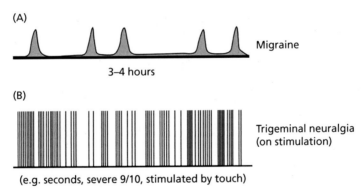

(A)

Migraine

3–4 hours

(B)

Trigeminal neuralgia (on stimulation)

(e.g. seconds, severe 9/10, stimulated by touch)

Fig. 5-5 (**A and B**) Representation of patterns of a patient's pain experience. Time detail has been entered below the diagram. In diagram (A), the patient describes severe recurrent and unstimulated pain, building in intensity and lasting for 3–4 hours before quickly dissipating (suggestive of migraine). In the second diagram (B), the patient describes e.g. severe pain that only lasts for a few seconds and is precipitated by touch, suggestive of trigeminal neuralgia.

are applicable to dental pain and should raise a flag when used. Thus, when listening to a patient's description, it is important not only to hear the descriptor but also to analyze what the descriptor means ("*What does that mean? What else do I need to know?*"). For example, when a patient reports sensitivity to sweets, a natural reaction of most clinicians is to jump to a clinical diagnosis. However, pain to sweetness is a very specific descriptor:

- *What does that mean?* It indicates three things: 1) the patient has a dental problem; 2) the tooth is vital; and 3) the dentin is exposed.
- *What else do I need to know?* The tooth is vital, so sensitivity testing of all teeth in the area is not indicated. What *is* necessary is to identify the

exposed dentin, which may be due to a number of causes.
- A similar analysis ("*What does that mean? What else do I need to know?*") should be made each time a descriptor is used.

Descriptors in the *McGill Pain Questionnaire* are arranged in groups (sensory, affective, evaluative and general). The following compilation of descriptors is adapted from those in the *McGill Pain Questionnaire*[54] but with other descriptors added.

Sensory descriptors

Sensory descriptors are important and explain how the pain feels to the patient. There are a large number of these; however, not all are specific for dental pain. More common descriptors of dental pain are high-lighted in italics. Sensory descriptors can be:

- Time related, e.g. flickering, quivering, pulsing, *throbbing*, beating, pounding
- Movement or space related, e.g. jumping, flashing, shooting, electric, jolting
- Describing a puncturing sensation, e.g. pricking, boring, drilling, *stabbing*
- Describing a cutting sensation, e.g. *sharp*, cutting, lacerating, splitting
- Describing a constricting sensation, e.g. pinching, pressing, gnawing, cramping, crushing, taut, vice-like
- Describing a pulling sensation, e.g. tugging, pulling, wrenching
- Describing perceived thermal sensations, e.g. hot, burning, scalding, searing, cold, freezing
- Describing abnormal sensation, e.g. numb, tingling, itching, smarting, stinging, irritated
- Describing non-acute pain, e.g. *dull, sore, hurting, aching, heavy, tender, unpleasant*
- Describing acute pain, e.g. *agonizing, dreadful, terrible, excruciating, severe, piercing, very bad*
- Describing presence, e.g. *constant, intermittent, sometimes, always.*

Sensory pain descriptors can also be broadly categorized as *bright*, sharp and superficial, or *dull*, less severe and more deeply seated. Pain can also be described as *spreading*, where the pain spreads slowly over a broad area, or *radiating*, where the pain spreads rapidly to another site. Orofacial pain can also be *referred* to another site, as happens in dental and muscular pains, or can *migrate* from site to site, as is common in trigeminal neuropathic orofacial pain.[56]

A second group of words describing pain are *affective descriptors*. Unlike sensory descriptors, these terms describe how the pain affects the patient. Patients can state how the pain makes them feel directly (e.g. *sick, nauseated, fearful, frightened, frustrated*), or communicate the same information by using descriptors (*tiring, exhausting, sickening, nauseating, frustrating*).

Special care has to be taken when managing patients who use affective descriptors that may have a psychological basis (e.g. *suffocating, punishing, cruel, vicious, grueling, killing, wretched, blinding, arduous, tormenting*). These patients may have a concomitant psychological problem.

A third group of descriptors are termed *evaluative*. These tend to indicate the intensity of pain. The *McGill Pain Questionnaire* lists the following evaluative descriptors: *annoying, troublesome, chronic, miserable, intense* and *unbearable.*

The descriptors the patient uses are extremely important when diagnosing orofacial pain. Special attention needs to be paid to them. As mentioned above, some of these descriptors are specific for dental pain, but others are not. For example:

- The words *dull* and *constant* used together commonly indicate muscle pain or occasionally sinusitis.
- *Itching* is often a descriptor for soft tissue or perio-dontal conditions.
- *Waves* may be a descriptor for pulpitis.
- *Throbbing, pressure, sharp, hurting, sore, aching* and *stabbing* are common dental descriptors
- Other descriptors, such as *punishing, cruel* or *vicious*, are more likely to be psychological descriptors (what the pain is doing to them).
- Special notice should be placed on the use of descriptors that are usually not used for describing dental pain. Descriptors including flashing. burning, jolting, movement and electric shock-like fit into this category. These descriptors are more likely to indicate a neurological cause.
- Some descriptors need qualification, e.g. the word *constant* (constant and severe, constant and dull, constantly there…).
- Some descriptors are cause and effect (*If this … then that*). These terms are helpful in assessing stimulated pain.
- Some descriptors are colloquial and specific to communities, countries or ethnic groups. They can vary from one group to another, and may need local interpretation.

It should be apparent from the above that patients can use a myriad of descriptors to describe orofacial pain. Assessing the meaning of descriptors and the patterns in which they are expressed provides a road map leading to an accurate diagnosis. Carefully listening to and recording descriptors used by the patient, and then analyzing reasons for these responses, are essential because many pain conditions exhibit patterns of symptoms that are mirrored in these descriptors. Pay particular attention when the manner in which the patient describes the pain and the descriptors they use do not *add up*. *The descriptors should fit the diagnosis.*

Chapter 6

Analyzing Patients in Pain – Observing Patients in Pain

Alex J. Moule and Tareq Al Ali

You can observe a lot just by watching. – Yogi Berra

Introduction

Early in the questioning of the patient it is necessary to establish the site of the pain. It is important to appreciate that patients can only report where they think the pain is. This location may not be the actual source of the pain. Pain can be referred from a distant source. Nevertheless, patients must be given an opportunity to describe, both in words and by physical demonstration, where they think the pain is located.

When trying to establish the site of pain, two questions to ask are:
Where is the pain?
Can you place your finger on where the pain is?

This chapter will describe the importance of asking a patient to physically demonstrate (describe) where the pain is rather than having them just tell you where it is. It is often helpful to record the pain diagnosis profile and location of the pain diagrammatically both intraorally and extraorally in the notes by shading or drawing in pain locations at the same time. This provides valuable documentation for later review. There are occasions, as happens with trigeminal neuropathic orofacial pain, where the orofacial pain can move to other parts of the body. There are also occasions where orofacial pain is a symptom of a more general condition where symptoms (e.g. numbness and muscle dysfunction) are experienced in parts of the body remote from the orofacial region. Thus, a full-body diagram is sometimes required (Fig. 6-1).

In addition to recording the patient's verbal descriptions, line drawings can also be used to characterize the type and severity of the pain (see Chapter 5). Constant mild pain, constant severe pain, stimulated pain, prolonged stimulated pain, pulsating pain and pain that has a daily pattern can all be illustrated diagrammatically and referred to later. These drawings are useful when dealing with complex cases, particularly when used with a visual analogue scale (VAS).

Certain pain conditions show distinctive patterns, which can be shown diagrammatically. Sinusitis, cluster headache, tension headache, migraine and TMD all have distinctive pain patterns that can be represented on a diagram (Fig. 6-2).

CAUTION: Pay close attention to any patient who has *a severe initial headache that continues to increase in severity,* or a headache with associated neurological signs or symptoms (e.g. facial numbness or visual disturbances). This could indicate the presence of an intracranial lesion. Immediate referral to a neurologist or an emergency medical center may be necessary.[58]

When questioned on the location of the site of their pain, a patient will verbally describe the site and then demonstrate or describe it non-verbally using their hands and fingers.[59] Note the manner in which the patient gestures while describing their pain. Patients may point to, touch or move fingers over a site. Many of these movements provide valuable diagnostic information. Some of these are described below. When observing the manner in which patients use physical actions to describe their pain, an astute clinician needs to ask themselves:

What does that action mean?
What more do I need to know?

Diagnosing Dental and Orofacial Pain: A Clinical Manual, First Edition. Edited by Alex J. Moule and M. Lamar Hicks.
© 2017 John Wiley & Sons, Ltd. Published 2017 by John Wiley & Sons, Ltd.
Companion website: www.wiley.com/go/moule/dental_and_orofacial_pain

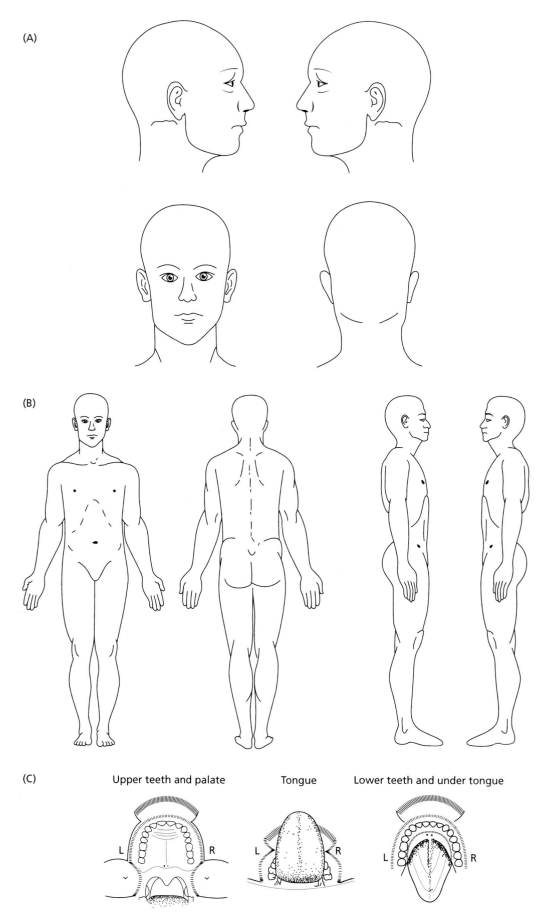

(A)

(B)

(C)   Upper teeth and palate   Tongue   Lower teeth and under tongue

Fig. 6-1 (A) Diagram of the head and neck on which the clinician or patient can draw the location of pain.
(B) Diagram of a body on which a clinician or patient can draw the location of pain.
(C) Diagram of teeth and intra-oral structures illustrating the palate, the dorsal and the undersurface of the tongue on which a clinician or patient can draw the location of pain.

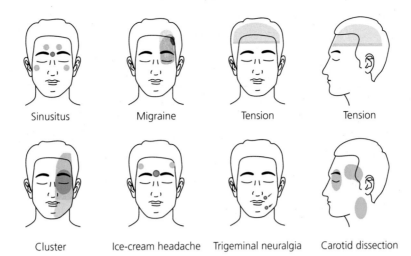

Sinusitus   Migraine   Tension   Tension

Cluster   Ice-cream headache   Trigeminal neuralgia   Carotid dissection

Fig. 6-2 Distribution of pain commonly seen in various conditions. Aadapted from: Lance, J.W. *Mechanism and Management of Headache*, 5th edn.[57]

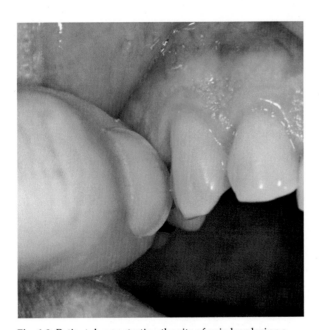

Fig. 6-3 Patient demonstrating the site of pain by placing a fingernail vertically between two teeth.

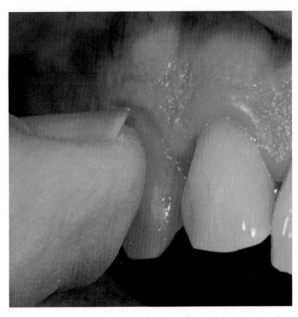

Fig. 6-4 Patient demonstrating their pain by scratching on the tooth close to the gingival margin with a fingernail.

Placing a fingernail vertically between two teeth

If a patient describes the location of pain by placing a fingernail vertically between two teeth (Fig. 6-3) (video 1), the action means that the pain is localized. It does not establish whether the discomfort is tooth or soft tissue related. Look initially for food impaction, then press on the interdental papilla with the back of a probe. Then ask:

Is this the type of pain you are feeling?

If the patient answers affirmatively, a soft tissue origin is highly likely. Cracked teeth and loose restorations can also be described in this way, but can be differentiated from soft tissue pain by pressing on the soft tissues as described above.

Moving a fingernail on a tooth

If a patient demonstrates pain by scratching or moving a fingernail over a tooth surface (Fig. 6-4) (video 2), this indicates that the pain is 1) localized, 2) tooth related and 3) can be provoked. Look initially for exposed dentin by scratching the tooth surface with a probe to try to reproduce the pain.

Placing a finger over the apex of a tooth

Patients who describe pain by pressing over the apex of a tooth (Fig. 6-5) (video 3) are demonstrating pain that is 1) localized and 2) usually of soft tissue origin. The position of the finger over the apex suggests that periapical pathology may be present. Another possibility is an ulcer.

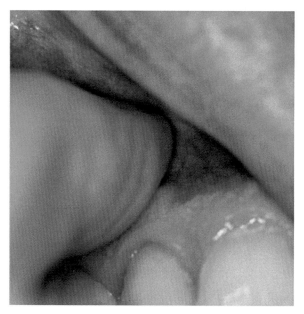

Fig. 6-5 Patient demonstrating their pain by pressing over a tooth apex.

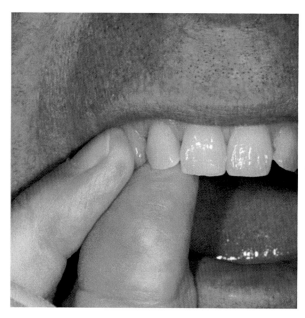

Fig. 6-7 Patient demonstrating their pain by holding and moving an individual tooth.

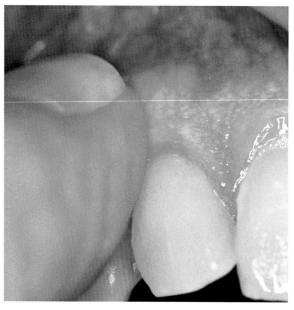

Fig. 6-6 Patient demonstrating their pain by pressing on the gingival margin.

Pressing on the gingival margin

If a patient indicates the pain is coming from the gingival margin (Fig. 6-6) (video 4), the pain is localized and probably of soft tissue origin. The position of the finger indicates that the pain is likely related to the periodontal inflammation rather than to periapical pathology. Check initially for a periodontal abscess or a vertical root fracture.

Rubbing a finger rapidly back and forth across attached gingiva

There is a difference between a patient *pressing* on the gingiva while moving a finger slowly versus *rubbing a finger rapidly back and forth* across the soft tissues.

Some patients may report soft tissue sensitivity that has a neuropathic or sensory nerve origin. Occasionally these patients describe the pain by moving a finger rapidly over a small segment of gingival margin or a dental papilla (video 5). The gingiva can be red and shiny due to the constant rubbing of a finger or the tongue over the site. If a soft tissue origin is confirmed and various local measures do not provide relief, the careful application of capsaicin cream (e.g. Zostrix®) may provide relief.

Holding one tooth

Patients can verbally describe toothache while at the same time holding and moving an individual tooth (Fig. 6-7) (video 6). This action indicates that their pain is 1) localized, 2) tooth related, and 3) involves the supporting tissues.

The subject tooth should be tested for vitality, percussion sensitivity and mobility. In the absence of obvious periapical involvement, check for periodontal problems, history of trauma, occlusal trauma or vertical root fracture. Patients who hold firmly onto a tooth after cold stimulation (to warm the tooth?) are experiencing localized dental pain.

Be very careful if the descriptors used by the patient seem unusual and cannot be explained. Trigeminal neuropathic orofacial facial pain and even some malignancies (e.g. maxillary adenocystic carcinoma) can present in this manner.

Holding or moving several teeth

Pain elicited by the movement of several teeth together or independently (Fig. 6-8) (video 7) indicates the pain is from supporting tissues and not from an individual tooth. There also may be pain to percussion. In the absence of frank periapical infection, this is not tooth pain. If there is a history of trauma, check for an alveolar fracture or fracture of the facial plate of bone (Fig. 6-9). *Pulp extirpation will not relieve this pain or any pain to percussion.*

Touching the side of the face

Much can be learned by the way a patient touches the side of the face when describing the location of pain. Of the many anatomical structures present in the orofacial region, including the skin, parotid gland, muscles, blood vessels, and facial and trigeminal nerves, any one of them can be responsible for pain.

A patient can indicate the location of pain on the side of the face in different positions and in different ways. Some patients are unable to locate pain to any specific area and may just cradle their face. Fortunately, most patients gesture with their hands and fingers in a distinctive manner that is helpful from a diagnostic point of view. For example, where and how the patient demonstrates pain by pressing on the side of the face, the number of fingers used and the manner in which they are applied to the face have great significance (Fig. 6-10).

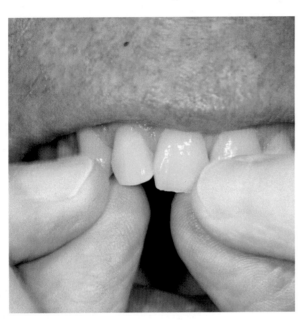

Fig. 6-8 Patient demonstrating their pain by movement of several teeth together or independently.

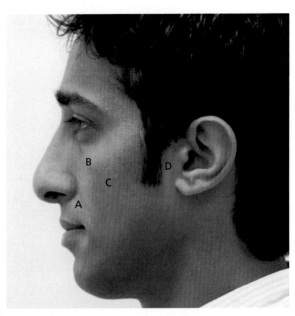

Fig. 6-10 Profile view of patient illustrating the four positions described below: (A) tenderness beside the nose; (B) tenderness immediately under the eye; (C) tenderness on the lateral border of the zygomatic arch just above the second premolar; (D) tenderness in front of the ear.

(A)

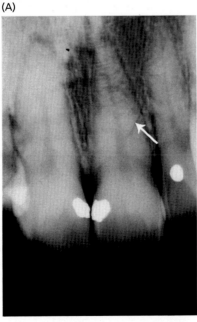

(B)

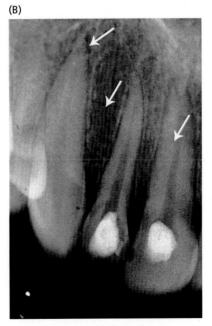

Fig. 6-9 Fractures in the facial plate of bone result in sensitivity to percussion of anterior teeth after impact trauma. In (A), there were multiple alveolar fractures (arrow) involving the entire buccal plate of bone. In (B), there appeared to be a single fracture running across the maxillary incisors and involving the canine tooth. Endodontic treatment did not relieve the pain and was contraindicated.

(A)

(B)

(C)

(D)

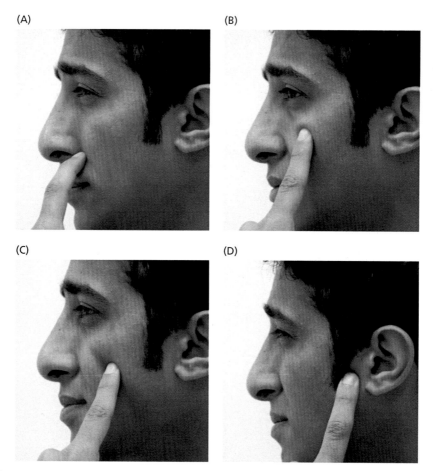

Fig. 6-11 Patient demonstrating tenderness or pain (A) beside the nose, (B) immediately under the eye, (C) on the lateral border of the zygomatic arch just above the maxillary second premolar and (D) in the temporomandibular joint area. Patients often use two fingers to demonstrate joint pain.

A. *Tenderness beside the nose*

Tenderness just lateral to the ala of the nose (Fig. 6-11) (video 8) is likely to be soft tissue pain related to periapical inflammation from a maxillary canine or lateral incisor. Other soft tissue pathoses (e.g. acne or an ulcer) need to be considered.

B. *Tenderness immediately under the eye*

Tenderness to palpation immediately under the eye in the area of the infra-orbital foramen (Fig. 6-11) (video 9) is often associated with maxillary sinusitis. Thus, screening for this possibility is indicated.

C. *Tenderness on the lateral border of the zygomatic arch above the second premolar*

Tenderness on the lateral border of the zygomatic arch immediately above the maxillary second premolar or first molar tooth (C) (Fig. 6-12) (video 10) suggests involvement of the anterior attachment of the masseter muscle. Confirm this by placing a finger firmly on the area of tenderness, and then asking the patient to clench. Increased tenderness during clenching will confirm masseter muscle involvement.

D. *Tenderness in front of the ear*

Pressing one or two fingers on the face immediately anterior to the tragus of the ear suggests

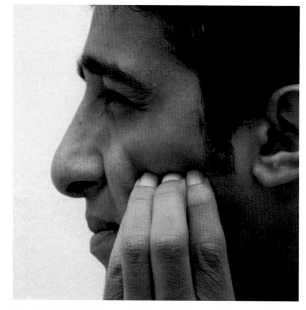

Fig. 6-12 Patient demonstrating pain by pressing several fingers on the body of the masseter.

arthralgia of the temporomandibular joint (Fig. 6-11) (video 11), especially if the fingers are moved in a circular motion and the patient moves their jaw.

Pressing under the maxilla

In the absence of obvious dental infection or other pathology, patients who describe pain by pressing in the middle of the face just under the maxilla (Fig. 6-12) are often describing masticatory muscle pain (video 12). This is particularly diagnostic if they move their fingers in a rotary motion. If parotid pathology is responsible, the area of tenderness will be located more posteriorly and the gland will be palpable. Important questions to ask, when developing a differential diagnosis or trying to explain this finding to a patient, are:

Is it painful if you press anywhere on the side of the face? Can you make it hurt if you press the side of the face?

NOTE: A patient can be assured of a non-dental origin by having them press into the body of the masseter and then clenching. Ask them whether the pain they are experiencing is the one they had experienced previously. Pain to palpation during clenching confirms a non-dental origin.

NOTE: Masticatory muscle pain can develop secondarily to other painful conditions and may become the main complaint. Therefore, a thorough investigation is required to exclude other causes.

Pressing on the body of the mandible with fingers in motion

If a patient describes pain by pressing on the side of their face with several fingers moving in a circular, palpating motion, they are probably massaging the masseter muscle (Fig. 6-13) (video 13). The patient

needs to be screened for muscle pain, especially if the movement is associated with a movement of the jaw.

Moving fingers in line under the mandible

A common complaint of patients with muscle spasm is that their *glands swell up under their jaw.* This is demonstrated by massaging the submandibular area with several fingers *in motion* and in line with the lower border of the mandible (Fig. 6-14) (video 14). These patients may have been prescribed several courses of antibiotics and may report that the pain disappears over time only to return days or weeks later. Patients who describe pain in this manner are likely to be describing pain associated with the posterior digastric muscle and should be screened for joint and muscle dysfunction.

Ask: *How long does it take for the antibiotics to work?*

If it is more than a few days, the relief is likely to be from the passage of time rather than from the antibiotics.

NOTE:
- If fingers are in motion when describing pain, the likelihood of a dental origin is diminished.
- When the patient moves their fingers independently to one another, pain is unlikely to be of dental origin.
- Patients who massage under the mandible with their fingers in line are usually palpating suprahyoid muscles (usually the posterior belly of the digastric muscle) and are describing pain from muscle dysfunction
- Salivary gland pathology rarely presents as just submandibular tenderness. When the tenderness does occur, it is usually intermittent and occurs shortly before or during eating.

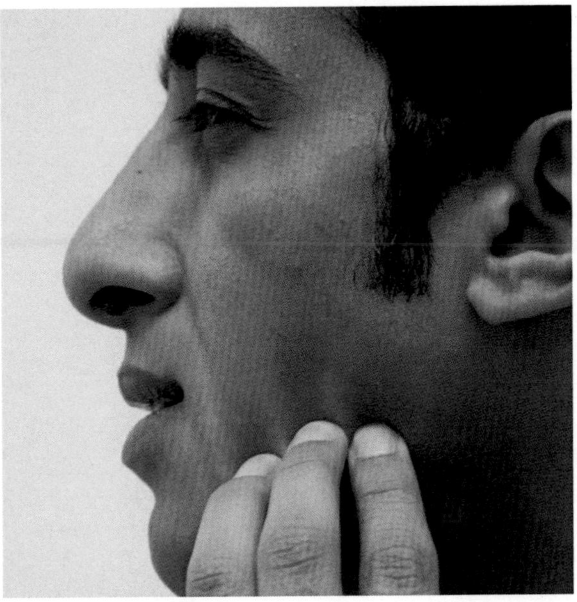

Fig. 6-13 Patient demonstrating pain by pressing on the body of the mandible. Muscle pain is most likely if the fingers are in motion, palpating the area.

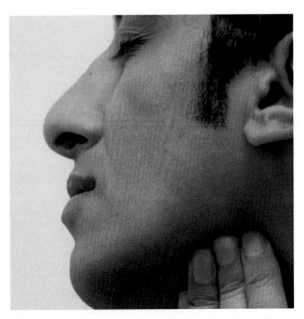

Fig. 6-14 Patient demonstrating pain by moving fingers in line under the mandible.

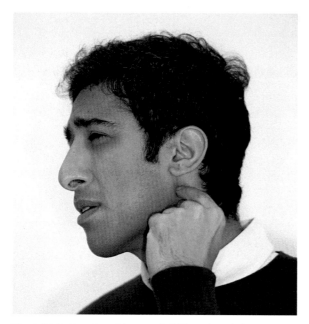

Fig. 6-15 Patient describing a painful lymph node by pointing at the node with a single finger.

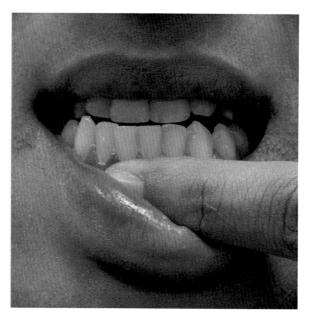

Fig. 6-16 Patient describing their pain by running a finger back and forth across the midline below the mandibular incisor tooth crowns.

When a patient describes pain from a lymph node, it is usually demonstrated with a single thumb or finger, or by picking up the gland between the thumb and finger in a more defined gesture (Fig. 6-15) (video 15).

Describing pain on all lower teeth by running a finger around the gingival margin

In the absence of frank periapical or periodontal pathology (e.g. acute necrotizing ulcerative gingivitis, HIV-P, periodontal or gingival abscesses), patients who complain that their gums are sore, or describe their pain by running their finger around the alveolar mucosa and gingiva (usually across the midline) (Fig. 6-16) (video 16), are describing pain associated with clenching. They often complain that the site of the pain is situated *half-way up the gum.*

NOTE: Of particular diagnostic importance is that the finger crosses the midline when the cause of the pain is being demonstrated. If a finger or hand used to describe orofacial pain crosses the midline, a non-dental problem is almost always the cause.

Describing pain with two hands

Patients with sinusitis, tension headaches, muscle pain and TMD may describe the location of the pain using two hands (video 17):

- If the pain is *bilateral and symmetrical,* screen for muscle pain and sinusitis.
Note: Bilateral pain is discussed below.
- If the pain is *unilateral* (Fig. 6-17) (video 18), check to see if the actions of describing the pain follow normal anatomical structures or pathways (e.g. nerves, blood vessels or muscle attachments). This will help in developing a differential diagnosis.

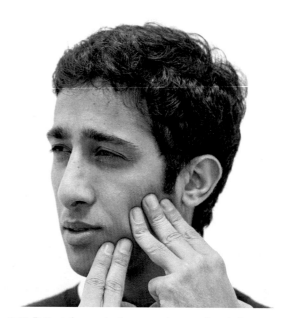

Fig. 6-17 Patient demonstrating masseter muscle pain by using two hands unilaterally.

- If the pain is *bilateral and asymmetrical,* consider anatomical explanations, but screen for neuropathic orofacial pain and psychosocial factors. Although rare, also consider the possibility that two unrelated causes exist for the pain.

NOTE: Be aware that some patients with persistent idiopathic facial pain use exaggerated two-handed gestures, which may be inconsistent with normal anatomy, to describe the distribution of their pain.

NOTE: Where two-handed descriptions of pain are not consistent with normal anatomy, screen for psychosomatic factors. Consider referring the patient for assessment by a specialist.

Bilateral pain

Once a patient states that their pain is bilateral, *all the rules change* because the pain is invariably not dental in origin. When investigating bilateral pain, consider the anatomic distribution of the pain and whether the pain is symmetrically situated on each side of the head (Fig. 6-18).

The three most common causes of bilateral facial pain are:

1. Muscle dysfunction (including referral of pain from the neck and shoulders) and temporomandibular joint arthralgia
2. Sinusitis (maxilla)
3. Neuropathic trigeminal orofacial pain.

Bilateral orofacial pain from other causes is rare. Central lesions rarely produce bilateral pain. Bilateral trigeminal neuralgia can occur, but is very uncommon, and the pain on each side is distinct and separate and may not involve the same division of the nerve on each side. Primary tumors or metastatic disease very rarely cause bilateral orofacial symptoms. In these rare instances, they are usually accompanied by other signs. In every pain diagnosis, always ask:

Do you get or have you had pain on the other side?

If a patient responds positively or with a statement such as, *"Yes, occasionally, but mostly it is on this side,"* it is indicative of a non-dental problem.

NOTE: Bilateral pain is almost always not dental pain, unless the cause of pain is in the midline.

Percussion pain on multiple teeth

In the absence of obvious periapical pathology, patients with pain on percussion of multiple teeth should be screened for clenching or occlusal trauma. A dental cause is highly unlikely. In the maxilla, maxillary sinus pathology has to be considered. Remember, however, that responses to percussion vary from patient to patient. What to some patients is a gentle tap on the tooth, is to others a severe blow. In order to assess pain on percussion, the response of the tooth in question should be compared to responses obtained from adjacent teeth and a corresponding tooth on the contralateral side. It is not sufficient to tap on one tooth and ask, *"Does this hurt?"* Almost always the answer will be *"yes."* It is best to assess responses to percussion testing by comparing them to the responses from other teeth:

I am going to tap on these teeth. Call this one number one, call this one number two, and call this one number three. Which one was more sensitive, one, two or three?

(A)   (B)

(C)   (D)

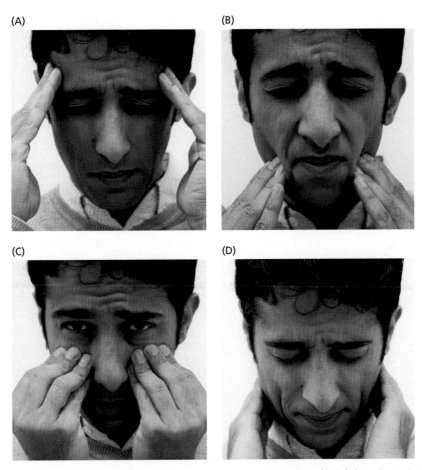

Fig. 6-18 Ways that symmetrical bilateral pain in the head and neck can be demonstrated: (A) bilateral pain in the temple, most likely from the temporalis muscles; (B) bilateral pain in the mandible, probably from the masseter muscle; (C) bilateral pain in the maxilla, from maxillary sinusitis; (D) bilateral pain centered in the posterior neck musculature.

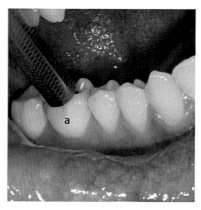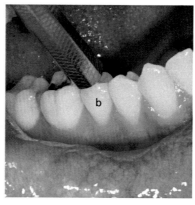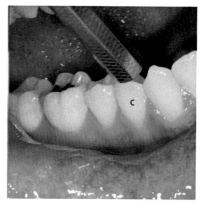

Fig. 6-19 Assessing the response to percussion. Determine the comparative response to a percussive blow on adjacent teeth. Always retest the teeth in a different order if any positive response is reported.

After the first cycle of percussion testing, repeat the testing in a different order (Fig. 6-19).

Some patients with trigeminal neuropathic facial pain or persistent idiopathic facial pain (PIFP) exhibit an exaggerated response to almost any stimulus. This makes an assessment of whether teeth are actually sensitive to percussion very difficult. In a small number of patients, percussion testing is not reliable.

Although the response to percussion must be reassessed or questioned when multiple teeth are sensitive, multiple tooth sensitivity can occur. As above, in the maxilla this can be due to a maxillary sinusitis. If teeth in both jaws are involved at the same time, screen for a clenching habit.

NOTE: Removal of a pulp (pulpectomy) from a vital anterior tooth will not relieve pain to biting or percussion unless the tooth is fractured or cracked.

Holding a hand on the side of the face

Most patients who describe the location of their pain by placing a hand on the side of their face or cradling their jaw(s) or face with a hand (Fig. 6-20) (video 19) are unable to localize the source of the pain. An appreciation of the severity of the pain can often be assessed by observing the facial expression and manner in which the patient drops their chin into their hand. The manner in which they cradle their face may indicate the severity of the pain. If the pain is deep and severe, dental pain from an acute pulpitis is suspected. Other patients may be describing muscle pain. Note whether the hand is moving when the pain is described. *If so, the possibility of dental causes is diminished.* If they report relief by placing their hand on the side of their face, they are most likely describing muscle pain and they should be screened for this.

Questions to ask: *Is the pain relieved by a hot shower or hot pack?*
Can you make the pain worse by pressing on the side of your face?

Similarly, if a patient reports relief from pain from a hot shower or a hot pack, then screen for muscle pain.

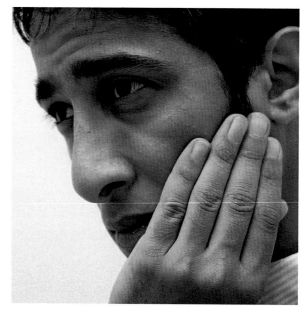

Fig. 6-20 Patient demonstrating the location of their pain by holding or cradling the side of the face.

Although a hot shower can provide some relief from the pain of a sinusitis, there are usually other associated signs and symptoms with this condition.

Complaining of inability to sleep on one side of the face

In the absence of frank periapical or other overt infection (e.g. unilateral maxillary sinusitis), if a patient reports that they cannot sleep on one side of their face, suspect muscle dysfunction, particularly a masseter muscle spasm. Thus, one of the screening questions for muscle pain is:

Does it hurt to sleep on that side of your face?

Pointing to an area, but reluctant to touch it

Patients suffering from trigeminal neuralgia can variously describe their pain experience. *Trigger points* can be present. Some patients may report that touching the trigger point sends a shooting pain up

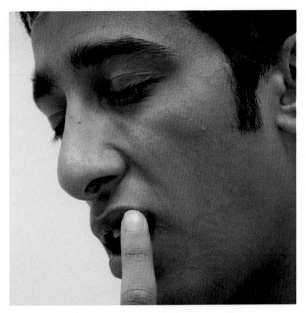

Fig. 6-21 Demonstration of a trigger point by lightly touching an area.

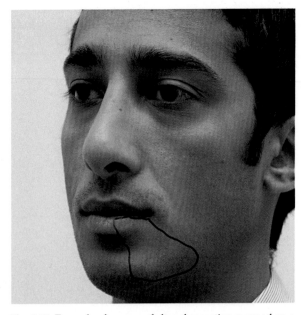

Fig. 6-22 Example of an area of altered sensation mapped on a patient's face and photographed.

the face or along the jaw (along one or more divisions of the trigeminal nerve). Although most patients are reluctant to touch the trigger point, others may very lightly touch the trigger to show its position (e.g. touching the corner of the mouth with the back of a fingernail) (Fig. 6-21) (video 20). They also may map out the distribution of the pain with one of their fingers and state, "*If I touch here, the pain shoots up here.*"

Some patients may use the other hand to show the distribution of the shooting pain once the trigger is activated. It is fairly obvious when pain from trigeminal neuralgia occurs. The patient often stops talking, the face may twitch and the eye may close slightly on the affected side. Some patients with trigeminal neuralgia insist that the pain is from a tooth. If a patient insists that the pain is dental, ask them to swallow with their teeth apart or touch the trigger point without touching any teeth (e.g. lifting the lip may help to confirm for the patient that the pain is not dental).

Any patient who describes shooting, electric shock-type pains should be asked the screening questions for trigeminal neuralgia. Other neuralgias also need to be considered (e.g. glossopharyngeal neuralgia, post-herpetic neuralgia).

Complaining of altered sensation

Numbness (anesthesia) and altered sensation (paresthesia) can occur as a symptom when mandibular premolar teeth and mandibular first molars are acutely infected. Be alert, however, for orofacial pain that is associated with altered sensation where no dental cause can be found. Although bacterial and viral infections are often implicated, the possibility of nerve damage, systemic disease or an intracranial lesion needs to be considered. Numbness or anesthesia

can occur in Bell's palsy (CN VII), which resolves in 6 to 8 weeks, and with a rare viral condition involving the mental nerve (branch of CN V).

Patients often indicate an area of altered sensation by rubbing or patting the affected area. When an area of lost or altered sensation is noted, the area should be mapped with a blunt probe. Then the area should be drawn on a diagram, or even marked directly on a patient's face and photographed (Fig. 6-22) (video 21). This enables the changes in the distribution of the numbness to be followed and documented. An increasing area of numbness is of concern and requires referral.

Altered sensation can be a sign of an impending herpes zoster (shingles) attack or Bell's palsy. When seen in conjunction with motor disturbances or altered sensation in other areas of the body (e.g. hands or feet), a differential diagnosis that includes multiple sclerosis and other neurological causes must be considered and referral is required.

NOTE: A patient may describe local areas of altered sensation by patting the side of the face or moving their fingers rapidly over the skin surface.

Describing pain in and around the eye

Pain in and around the eye (Fig. 6-23) can be caused by a number of conditions. Migraine headache, sinus conditions including ethmoid sinusitis, eye problems, trauma, cluster headaches and carotid dissection are some of the possibilities.

When assessing the patient who describes pain in or around the eye, note any previous history of the complaint and associated signs and symptoms, especially any visual disturbances. Migraine headaches

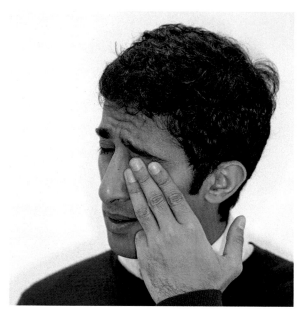

Fig. 6-23 Demonstration of orofacial pain in and around the eye. Note whether the patient is describing general pain that includes the eye or whether the pain is in or behind the eye.

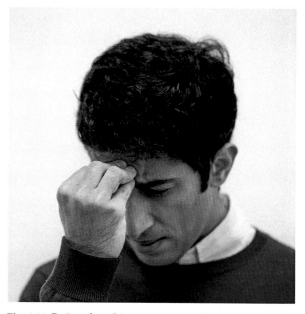

Fig. 6-24 Patient describing pain centered between the eyes. Frontal or ethmoid sinusitis and referred muscle pain are common causes.

often occur behind the eye and can involve blurring of vision or the presence of an aura. Most patients are aware of migraine. Cluster headache is usually associated with Horner's syndrome (ptosis and miosis). Headache pain and visual disturbances may be a sign of giant cell arteritis. Carotid dissection, a life-threatening condition, must be considered when there is an initial episode of severe eye pain with concomitant Horner's syndrome.

Urgent referral is critical for any patient where the cause of pain that occurs in or around the eye along with any visual disturbances cannot be quickly determined. Upon referral, central lesions will need to be excluded.

Describing pain between the eyes

Patients with frontal or ethmoid sinus conditions can present with pain between the eyes (Fig. 6-24). It is common, however, for pain from the sternocleido-mastoid muscle to also be referred to this site. Pain between the eyes is not of dental origin.

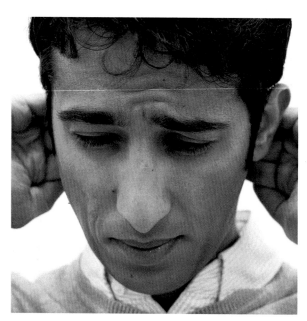

Fig. 6-25 Note whether the hand or fingers stray from the distribution of the trigeminal nerve. If they do, a dental cause is unlikely. If the pain is bilateral, it is not dental pain.

Describing pain around the base of the skull

If a patient presents for facial pain diagnosis, but also states that bilateral pain is present around the base of the skull (Fig. 6-25) or in a band around the head, screen for tension headache and muscle dysfunction.

If the pain is *unilateral,* screen for cervicogenic pain, neck or shoulder problems and postural problems common in the workplace. Carefully observe when a patient describes their pain as to whether the hand or fingers stray from the distribution of the trigeminal nerve (video 22). Note also whether the hand movement is associated with movement of the neck or jaw. Except for acute infections, these patients are unlikely to be describing pain of dental origin. Remember, however, that the auriculo-temporal branch of the mandibular division of the trigeminal nerve supplies sensory innovation around and behind the ear and that it is common for mandibular molar tooth pain to be referred to this area.

NOTE: Dental pain is almost always referred to a branch of the maxillary or mandibular division of the trigeminal nerve. Where a patient's pain description

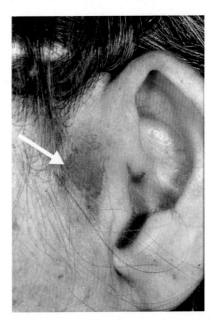

Fig. 6-26 Patient with severe orofacial pain who has demonstrated the pain by constantly rubbing the area directly over the TMJ joint (arrow). Screening questions and testing will establish whether the pain is from the joint or referred from another site.

involves sites outside the distribution of this nerve, the complaint is rarely of dental origin.

NOTE: Patients may develop facial muscle pain as a secondary problem due to the stress of an underlying dental or non-dental problem. The muscle pain can then become the patient's chief complaint. Treatment of the facial muscle pain may need to occur first before an accurate diagnosis of the underlying problem can be made. Patients with chronic medical conditions, such as chronic fatigue, often develop secondary facial muscle and joint pain.

In diagnosing orofacial pain, it is as important to watch the body language of the patient and observe how they physically demonstrate (describe) where the pain is, as well as having them verbally tell you where it is. Often the manner in which patients physically describe their pain (Fig. 6-26) governs the screening questions and testing that will be used to establish a diagnosis.

Chapter 7

Analyzing Patients in Pain – Associations with Cold and Heat

Alex J. Moule and M. Lamar Hicks

Introduction

In the previous chapter, the importance of listening to a patient's use of descriptors when answering initial questions (e.g. *What sort of pain are you having?*) was emphasized, as was the need to establish whether there was any history of thermal sensitivity early in the history-taking.

With all history-taking it is important not only to know what question to ask (*What should I ask?*), but to listen and analyze the response (*What does that answer mean? What else do I need to know?*). Previously, type of analysis was discussed regarding a history of sensitivity to sweetness (i.e. the tooth is vital; dentin is exposed). This chapter reviews the patient's descriptions of orofacial pain which are associated with temperature changes in the same manner.

Temperature sensitivity

Patients with orofacial pain from a dental cause often report sensitivity to thermal changes. Even if this is not initially reported, it is important to ask whether there has been such a history, as the answer often helps discriminate between pain of dental origin and pain from non-dental causes.

Responses to questioning can often be broken down into sub-sets that help with diagnosis. This is especially true with reactions to thermal stimuli. A number of scenarios are possible, all of which have different diagnostic importance. These are discussed below:

- Pain to cold
- Bilateral sensitivity to cold
- Pain to cold relieved by heat
- Pain to heat
- Pain to heat relieved by cold
- Delayed response to heat
- Unexplained sensitivity to cold
- Pain to cold and biting on a posterior tooth
- Pain when the patient goes out into the cold
- Pain to swallowing cold foods or drinks (ice cream headache)
- Pain relieved by placement of hand on side of face or by hot pack or hot shower.

Pain to cold

An intra-oral pain reaction to a cold stimulus indicates that the problem is dental, almost without exception, and that the pulp is vital. The status of the pulp is difficult to determine from one descriptor alone; however, the severity of the response and the duration of the sensation are factors that help in pulpal diagnosis. Most teeth that are only sensitive to cold are suffering from reversible pulpitis. If the sensitivity is not severe or prolonged, the offending tooth can be identified and the cause eliminated; only conservative treatment measures are usually necessary.

Bilateral sensitivity to cold

Other than general sensitivity due to exposed dentin, it is unusual for a patient to have two teeth that respond abnormally to cold, particularly bilateral teeth that respond at the same time. However, it could happen if a patient has multiple carious teeth or bilateral maxillary sinusitis. In both these situations, other signs are present.

Bilateral sensitivity to cold is usually due to stimulation of exposed dentin, or transmission of thermal stimulation through very thin enamel in teeth that

Diagnosing Dental and Orofacial Pain: A Clinical Manual, First Edition. Edited by Alex J. Moule and M. Lamar Hicks.
© 2017 John Wiley & Sons, Ltd. Published 2017 by John Wiley & Sons, Ltd.
Companion website: www.wiley.com/go/moule/dental_and_orofacial_pain

have suffered erosion, abrasion or attrition. Many patients who complain of bilateral pain to cold have already assessed that they have sensitive teeth. Many have been or are being treated with dentin desensitizing agents and desensitizing toothpastes. Sometimes, the difficulty is convincing new patients that the pain is related to exposed dentin. Stimulating the teeth by blowing air over the surface of the suspected tooth and then confirming an area of exposed and sensitive tooth structure with a probe are usually all that is required. As the pain is due to fluid movement in dentinal tubules, teeth should be tested "wet" without previous drying.

Pain to cold relieved by heat

As a general rule, teeth that are sensitive to cold, but relieved by heat, are far less likely to have irreversible pulpitis than teeth exhibiting a painful response to heat that is relieved by cold. The pulpal diagnosis can usually be determined from the history and the severity of the response (see Chapter 12). Thus, the problem for the clinician is only to identify the tooth involved. History provides the diagnosis; testing identifies the tooth in question.

Cold-sensitive teeth can be easily identified with the use of ice water under rubber dam isolation, isolating and testing each tooth individually. Testing should commence with the most posterior tooth in the quadrant. The severity of the pain is determined by assessing the patient's response and noting how long the pain lingers after the cold stimulus is removed.

The application of very cold water on individual teeth under rubber dam isolation is more accurate in identifying temperature-sensitive teeth than using cold pulp testing devices such as sprays and carbon dioxide snow, as these methods often only test a small section of a tooth. Some temperature-sensitive cracked teeth do not respond in a predictable manner unless the cold water actually flows over and into the crack.

Asking the question: *Is it ouch and gone type pain?* (suggesting reversible changes in the pulp) or: *Is it ouch and stay type pain?* (suggesting irreversible changes) is a useful method of assisting the patient to explain their response to thermal stimuli.

Also the question: *Was that the type of pain that you have been experiencing?* can help to confirm the identity of the responsive tooth. Even if a patient responds affirmatively to this question, all teeth in the arch (and often on that side) should still be tested to ensure the accuracy of the diagnosis:

- With few exceptions, sensitivity to cold is an indicator that the pain problem is tooth related.
- Sensitivity to cold indicates that there is vital tissue in the root canal.
- There is no justification for giving antibiotics to a patient with temperature-sensitive teeth, especially if there is a history of sensitivity to cold.

Pain to heat

There are no evidence-based data regarding the relationship between pulpitis and responses to thermal stimulation. Nevertheless, it would appear that in the early stages of pulpitis, teeth are sensitive first to cold stimulation. As inflammation develops, teeth can become sensitive to both cold and heat. In the later stages of pulpitis, heat sensitivity predominates. Teeth that are sensitive only to heat are more likely to have an irreversible pulpitis

Pain to heat relieved by cold

Patients who report severe pain from heat are more likely to have teeth with irreversible pulpitis than patients who report pain only to cold. In the later stages of pulpitis, teeth can become acutely sensitive to heat. So much so that patients may hold cold water in their mouth or suck on ice cubes in an attempt to relieve pain where the mouth temperature is sufficient to produce the pain (Fig. 7-1). These patients have an irreversibly inflamed pulp.

When a patient presents these signs and symptoms, and if the diagnosis is not clear, methodical testing of all teeth on that side with cold spray and a cotton pellet will identify the aching tooth. Relief of pain establishes a probable diagnosis. Repeating the procedure confirms the diagnosis.

A delayed response to heat

In the late stages of pulpal inflammation, teeth may no longer respond to cold stimuli or show immediately to heat, but may exhibit a *delayed* strong response to heat. This is a sign of irreversible

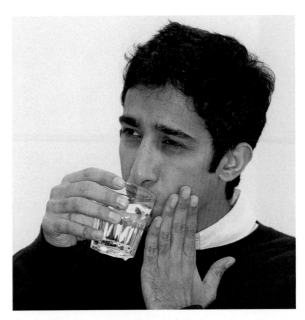

Fig. 7-1 Patients who present in dental pain, and who report that the pain is relieved by cold water or ice, are describing acute pulpitis.

pulpitis. Clinically many of these teeth exhibit non-vital tissue in the coronal pulp chamber.

NOTE: If a history of delayed pain occurring after the application of heat is obtained, identify the aching tooth by testing with hot water under rubber dam (see Chapter 11). It may be necessary to leave the hot water on each tooth for five to ten seconds. To avoid confusion, it is often better to delay testing the adjacent tooth for at least a minute until the pain has dissipated in order to assess the response.

Occasionally, pain can be initiated by the application of heat, but it is difficult to assess whether the source of the pain is from one or the other of two adjacent teeth. Analyzing the reason for responses to testing can greatly assist in the diagnostic process. Immediate re-testing with cold by holding a cold-sprayed cotton pellet on the suspected tooth for a few seconds can assist in diagnosis (Fig. 7-2):

- In many cases, delayed pain to heat can be reversed by applying cold to the offending tooth. If this occurs, it is likely to be the tooth in question. The origin of the pain can be confirmed by repeating the procedure
- Application of cold may produce a slight or no response and does not change the character of the pain. If this occurs, the cold-tested tooth is not the one involved.
- Rarely, application of cold to the involved tooth will dramatically increase the severity of the pain. If this occurs this is likely to be the tooth in question.

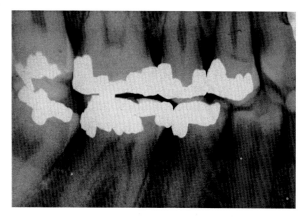

Fig. 7-2 Radiograph of a patient who presented with a history of severe but delayed pain when drinking hot beverages. The mandibular right second molar and then the first molar tooth were tested with hot water under rubber dam isolation. Severe pain resulted, but as both teeth had been tested before the pain started, the identity of the tooth in question was not clear. Testing with cold spray produced a very slight response on the first molar but immediately relieved the pain on the second molar. The first molar was then re-tested separately, first with heat and then immediately with cold spray to relieve the pain. The tooth was then endodontically treated.

Being able to change the character of a patient's pain by alternating hot and cold stimuli is helpful in identifying heat-sensitive teeth. In rare situations, it may be necessary to bring the patient back when the pain has completely subsided. Then carry out testing on only one tooth at a time. If this is the case, teeth can be tested individually to assess their response to heat, with a period of waiting between each test. Re-application of cold spray to reverse the pain responses can then be used to reconfirm the identity of the heat-sensitive tooth.

NOTE: In many cases, delayed pain to heat can be reversed by applying cold to the offending tooth. If this occurs, the identity of the tooth is confirmed. This is especially useful in diagnosing referred pain where the site and source of the pain are different.

Unexplained sensitivity to cold on posterior teeth

Many conditions can result in a patient reporting an increased sensitivity to cold in a vital tooth, including a recent restoration, occlusal trauma, exposed dentine, caries, a loose restoration or a crack in a tooth. It is unlikely, however, that the pulp in an intact restored tooth will suddenly become responsive to thermal changes over time, unless the environment in which it is situated has changed. Examples of these changes are caries, cracking, occlusal trauma and micro-leakage or leakage at the crown margins. It is important therefore to assess the possible cause of the pain, as well as to identify and treat the pain itself. The most likely cause of unexplained sensitivity to cold in a posterior tooth is the existence of a crack. In assessing these teeth, the factors to consider are:

Why has this tooth suddenly become sensitive to thermal changes?
What has changed to make this tooth now sensitive to thermal changes?

In some patients with rhinosinusitis, maxillary molar teeth can be sensitive to cold. In some but not all of these patients, the pain is intensified with postural change.

Root-filled teeth sensitive to cold

Patients sometimes report that a root-filled tooth is, or has become, sensitive to cold. Root-filled teeth very rarely become sensitive to cold stimulation. In almost all cases, patients are reporting sensitivity *in an adjacent tooth*. Mistakes occur if practitioners take the patient's description at face value. Sensitivity to cold can occur in a root-filled tooth due to stimulation of vital pulp tissue in an unprepared canal. Isolating each tooth on the one side (including the root-filled tooth) and testing with hot

(A)

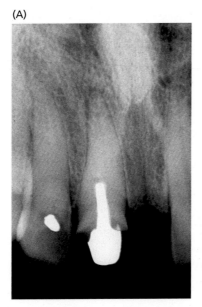

(B)

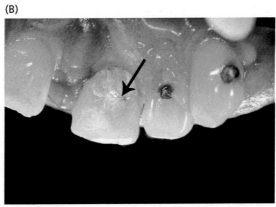

Fig. 7-3 Periapical radiograph of an acutely temperature-sensitive calcified tooth (A). A post was recently placed, and the tooth restored with an acrylic temporary crown. The post was exposed to the oral environment (arrow) (B), leading to transfer of thermal stimuli to a vital pulp in the calcified root canal.

or cold water under rubber dam isolation is a rapid way to confirm the identity of (and to convince the patient of the identity of) the thermally sensitive tooth. If thermal sensitivity is confirmed in a root-filled molar tooth, access into the pulp chamber without local anesthetic (Fig. 7-2) and investigation of the canal floor will usually confirm the presence of the canal. It also helps to confirm to a patient why further root canal treatment is required. Cone beam computed tomography (CBCT) may be helpful in these cases to identify the presence of an uninstrumented canal.

An unprepared canal is not the only cause of temperature sensitivity in a previously root-treated tooth. Rarely, the presence of a metallic root material (e.g. a silver point, broken file or metallic carrier) that is in contact with a metallic filling can result in thermal stimulation of remaining vital pulp or periodontal tissues. A similar situation can occur where a metallic core is in contact with a separated file or against vital tissue in a calcified canal that has not been located (Fig. 7-3).

Pain when the patient goes out into the cold

Patients can report that they get facial pain when they *"go out in the cold."* This symptom may be either volunteered by patients or elicited by questioning. The important question to ask here is:

Is this with your mouth open or your mouth closed?

(a) If a patient experiences this pain with their mouth closed, then the pain is not dental in origin. The most common cause is masseter spasm or other facial muscle spasm. Some of these patients often report that they cannot drive a car with the air conditioning on or with the window open, go into a refrigerated area in the supermarket or a cold room at work, or go outside on a cold or windy day.

(b) If the pain is elicited with the mouth open (drawing in a breath), then a dental problem is more likely the cause. In these cases, tooth identification can usually be made quickly by the use of cold water under rubber dam (see Chapter 11).

NOTE: If a patient presents with a complaint of pain when going out in the cold, establish whether the pain is felt with the mouth closed or open.

Pain to swallowing cold foods or drinks (ice cream headache)

Some patients experience intense brief stabbing head pain a few seconds after eating something cold, particularly if it is eaten quickly. Ice cream headaches (brain freeze, spenopalatine ganglionneuralgia) are experienced by males and females of all ages, and occur when the *patient eats something cold*. They are most likely to occur on a hot day or after exercise. The pain develops in the center of the forehead supra-orbitally, below the eyebrows, on the side of the fore-head or on the anterior part of the temple. *There is usually a refractory period of ten to fifteen seconds* before the onset of pain. The pain lasts for only seconds but in some persons can be extreme. The pain is thought to be related to cooling and subsequent vasoconstriction when cold material contacts the palate.

Pain relieved by hot pack or hot shower, or by placement of hand on side of face

Patients with facial muscle spasm can often obtain relief from symptoms by the application of heat to that side of the face. This relief is of diagnostic importance and indicates that a tooth is not the cause of the discomfort. Muscle palpation will usually reveal tenderness in the masseter muscle.

Patients who have cervicogenic headache pain also gain relief from the application of heat. This fact is helpful when diagnosing long-term orofacial pain. If the patient wakes with pain, but the pain is much better after a hot shower, the pain is likely to be cervicogenic in origin and the patient may benefit from referral to a physical therapist (physiotherapist). Patients who receive relief in the anterior face from taking a hot shower may alternatively be suffering from sinusitis.

Ask: *Do you get any relief by placing heat on the side of the face?*

Tooth pain is not relieved by the application of heat to the side of the face. Muscle pain can be.
Do you get any relief from a hot shower?

Toothache is not relieved by a hot shower.

While an intra-oral reaction to thermal stimuli is usually associated with pain of dental origin, there are a number of very different scenarios associated with a patient's pain response to thermal stimulation, not all of which are tooth related. Responses to questioning often need to be broken down to sub-sets that help with diagnosis. With all history taking, it is important to know what questions to ask, and then to listen and analyze the response.

Chapter 8

Analyzing Pain Descriptions – Pain on Biting or Eating and Other Considerations

Alex J. Moule and M. Lamar Hicks

Introduction

When a patient complains of pain on biting, the practitioner must understand what the patient means when they use the term "biting" or another similar term. When the discomfort or pain occurs is also important. Whether the discomfort starts before eating, at the commencement of or during chewing, or after eating must be determined. Time of onset has significance.

Pain on biting or chewing can originate from the temporomandibular joints, muscles of mastication, teeth or soft tissues of the oral cavity. The pain can variously be described as sharp, dull or electric shock-like. It can be fleeting, brief or prolonged. Diagnosis is easier and more accurate when attention is focused on the patient's description, the descriptors used, and the reported location and intensity of the pain. From a diagnostic perspective and for treatment purposes, it is necessary to distinguish between pains produced by biting, chewing and/or eating. A number of different scenarios follow in which pain is produced during functioning of the jaws. The following are described in this chapter:

- pain on biting
- pain in vital posterior teeth on biting
- biting pain in vital anterior teeth
- pain on eating
- pain before eating
- pain at the commencement of chewing
- pain when chewing
- pain after eating

- pain on biting accompanied by a bad taste
- pain relieved by biting
- biting pain after a crown is placed on a root canal-filled tooth.

Pain on biting

When a patient describes pain on biting it is suggestive of pain from a single tooth. The most common cause is a periapical infection associated with a tooth with a necrotic pulp. These teeth are relatively easy to diagnose. The patient can identify the tooth; the tooth is tender to percussion; there is a negative response to pulp sensibility testing; there may be a previous history of pulpitis; and frequently there are associated radiographic changes. The tooth can feel "high". Some teeth can be extremely sensitive to percussion or even touching. At other times, the patient simply avoids the tooth and states that it is a *little sore* if they bite on it. An ache that is prolonged after a biting event in a tooth that is also sore to bite on is a characteristic sign of periapical pathosis.

Teeth in traumatic occlusion can be sensitive to biting forces. In particular, teeth that have been recently restored may become sensitive to normal biting pressures, presenting usually as being *sore to bite on* rather than acutely painful. Unless the tooth is root canal treated, responses to pulp testing are normal. Teeth may or may not be overly sensitive to percussion. Some teeth are in traumatic occlusion only over a small range of a complete excursive movement. Careful testing with articulating paper will usually identify the exact location or spot of the

Diagnosing Dental and Orofacial Pain: A Clinical Manual, First Edition. Edited by Alex J. Moule and M. Lamar Hicks.
© 2017 John Wiley & Sons, Ltd. Published 2017 by John Wiley & Sons, Ltd.
Companion website: www.wiley.com/go/moule/dental_and_orofacial_pain

traumatic interference. Placing a finger on the buccal aspect of the interproximal surface of the tooth in question and asking the patient to squeeze and grind the teeth together will usually confirm the presence of an occlusal interference in an excursive movement, as the tooth will move slightly. Slight tooth mobility or noticeable movement of the tooth during an excursive movement confirms the diagnosis. Because tooth mobility can mask the identification of an occlusal interference, stabilizing the buccal surface of the tooth with a finger during the examination may be necessary to identify the interference. A single tooth with a crown can often be the cause of biting pain due to an occlusal interference that has developed over time.

Teeth with a history of a luxation injury or crown fracture can present with transient biting pain. Once a displaced tooth is repositioned, splinted and the occlusion adjusted, or the exposed dentin covered on a coronal fracture, the pain generally subsides once the acute phase is over. Occasionally, adult patients who suffer concussive blows to anterior teeth experience pain on biting or percussion for many months. Although unusual, the presence of a minor alveolar fracture must be considered. Patients who suffer severe indirect trauma where the maxillary and mandibular teeth are brought into contact with great force can suffer multiple cracked teeth, some of which may be difficult to detect.

Patients can report sharp, electric shock-like pain when touching a single tooth. In the absence of an obvious dental pathosis, the possibility of a dental trigger for trigeminal neuralgia should be considered. The exceedingly sharp pain in these cases is similar to *but not the same as* that experienced in a cracked tooth. The pain is initiated by only a slight touch. A cracked tooth usually requires a firm biting force or a firm percussive blow during diagnostic testing to initiate the pain. Pulp sensibility testing is required to rule out pulpal or periapical pathosis.

Pain in vital posterior teeth on biting

Although teeth in the late stages of irreversible pulpitis can occasionally respond ambivalently to vitality testing and be percussion sensitive, almost all *vital posterior teeth that are sensitive to biting forces* are cracked. The pain profile in these patients is one of an occasional unexpected sharp pain on biting, particularly when something small and hard is between the teeth. The tooth can be sensitive to cold fluids. While thermal and biting sensitivity in a vital cracked molar tooth can be eliminated by pulp extirpation, it is imperative that the cause of the discomfort be ascertained first. Pulp extirpation is inappropriate in a number of other situations where vital teeth are sensitive to percussion or biting. These include maxillary sinusitis, a clenching habit, occlusal trauma and trigeminal neuralgia. A thorough discussion of cracked teeth is found in Chapter 13.

Biting pain in vital anterior teeth

In contrast to posterior teeth, the situation in anterior teeth is entirely different. *If a vital anterior tooth is sensitive to biting pressure, then it is unlikely that removal of the pulp will have an effect on the pain.* Unless there is an obvious cause such as a fracture or crack, clinicians should be wary of any patient who reports pain on biting in a vital anterior tooth. The pain is likely to be of non-dental origin. Extirpation of the pulp is contraindicated and, if done, may only exacerbate the patient's problem. Although occlusal trauma and bony fractures have to be considered, neuropathic facial pain (atypical odontalgia, phantom tooth pain) can present in this manner.

Pain on eating

Pain on eating is a descriptor that can be interpreted as pain on biting *or* pain on chewing. As discussed below, patients who report pain on eating require further questioning. The pain may be from any of a large number of sources both in and outside the oral cavity. These include the tooth (e.g. a cracked tooth or exposed dentin), the tooth-supporting tissues (e.g. periapical pathosis), masticatory muscles, the temporomandibular joint, salivary gland dysfunction, impacted food, soft tissue pathoses, or ulcerations or cranial arteritis (rare). In each of these, the manner in which the patient describes the pain and the descriptors used are different. If observed and interpreted correctly, diagnosis is reasonably easy.

Pain before eating

Submandibular pain and eating are frequently associated with a pathosis of the submandibular gland (e.g. stenosis of the duct). Other signs and symptoms are invariably present and include localized submandibular pain and swelling in the floor of the mouth. Submandibular gland pain usually commences just *before* eating.

Pain at the commencement of chewing

Cramping of muscles that gradually develops during exercise, but eases when the muscles are rested, is called claudication. Jaw claudication, which develops as a result of inflammatory stenosis of the branches of the maxillary artery, is a sign of giant cell arteritis (GCA). It usually involves the jaw muscles, but also can involve the tongue or throat. It may be mistaken for temporomandibular joint dysfunction (TMD). This is a serious condition that requires immediate referral, particularly if visual disturbances are also present. GCA can result in infarct in the affected cranial artery. If the posterior ciliary artery is involved, the permanent blindness in the affected eye usually is followed a few weeks later by blindness in the other one. If you are unsure of a diagnosis of TMD, assess the onset of symptoms and ask the patient if they have suffered visual disturbances, especially temporary loss of vision.

Pain when chewing

The location and type of pain are helpful diagnostic clues for the diagnosis of pain on chewing. The pain can present in the jaw and face extraorally or intraorally in teeth. The pain can be sharp or dull.

Dull extra-oral pain during chewing is almost always of muscle origin. The masseter muscle may show tenderness and be hypertrophied. Jaw claudication, although rare, must be considered. Avoidance of chewing on one side is a sign of muscle dysfunction. The pain can usually be relieved with a hot pack.

Temporomandibular joint pain, if present, can be sharp or dull depending on the pathosis. If the joint is inflamed, the patient will be able to locate this easily by pressing externally on the joint in front of the tragus of the ear, while opening and closing. There will usually be a history of TMD. Occasionally, however, patients present with pain on chewing as their initial complaint after a recent traumatic injury of the TMJ, gum chewing or yawning too widely. Diagnosis can be made by pressing on the joints and asking the patients to open and close, simulating a chewing action. A thorough examination of the TMJ and palpation of the muscles of mastication should routinely be performed for patients presenting with orofacial pain. Patients may also present complaining of *toothache* when, in fact, the problem is of muscular or joint origin.

Patients with severely decayed teeth can experience pain on chewing due to food impaction into open defects in hard and soft tissues and between the teeth. This is usually easy to localize. Pain during eating can also be caused by a variety of easily identified soft tissue pathological conditions (e.g. the ulcers or vesicles of HSV infection, the mucocutaneous lesions of primary herpetic stomatitis, and erosive or ulcerative lesions such as those produced by lichen planus).

Pain after eating

Pain after eating can result from a number of causes, the most common of which is muscle dysfunction. Excluding trismus and acute muscle trauma, pain after eating is usually characterized as a dull pain that develops after eating and continues for some time. The muscles of mastication are usually sore to palpation. Pain after eating from a temporomandibular joint cause is usually noticed first while eating and is often more acute at the time of chewing. Patients avoid wide mouth opening as a protective or guarding mechanism and may restrict their food intake to avoid eating discomfort.

Pain on biting accompanied by a bad taste

Although pain and bad taste during biting may be associated with food impaction and a history of dental problems, the chief complaint is usually associated with a vertical root fracture or occasionally a loose restoration. Other intraoral dental causes are rare and usually obvious when they are present. If the patient can *initiate* the bad taste by sucking on a tooth, an intraoral cause should be considered. Medications used to treat cancer, gastric reflux and central lesions involving cranial nerve VII also can cause displeasing alterations in taste.[60] Patients with burning mouth syndrome (BMS) can have a constant bad taste in their mouth. Obviously, periodontal or restorative treatment will not relieve this annoying symptom. Other signs and symptoms of BMS include stress and xerostomia. When considering BMS, it is important to rule out obvious dental pathology before referring the patient to an oral medicine specialist for assessment and treatment. Medication and stress management are often prescribed.

Pain relieved by biting

Biting on teeth in the early stages of periapical inflammation can help relieve pain. Additionally, patients with sinusitis can also obtain pain relief by clenching their teeth. These patients may demonstrate their uncomfortable feeling associated with the maxillary molar teeth by tapping their teeth together. They may also state that their maxillary teeth feel strange or *woody*.

Biting pain after a crown is placed on a root canal-filled tooth

Some patients may present with a complaint that an endodontically treated tooth has become sensitive to biting. The question to ask these patients is:

Was your tooth comfortable before the crown was placed?

If the tooth became symptomatic after the crown was placed, the full coverage restoration has to be regarded as the cause of the pain. Careful examination may reveal that the crown is slightly high when the patient moves from centric occlusion into an excursive movement. As previously discussed, assessment for this occlusal discrepancy is done by placing a finger on the embrasure, touching the new crown and the adjacent tooth, and asking the patient to close their teeth together and grind. If the crown moves independently of the other teeth during this maneuver, there is an occlusal interference present that requires adjustment. This movement may be minor. When the patient has been uncomfortable for some time, a second adjustment a few days later may be necessary for the tooth to slowly assume a completely normal status. In more extreme situations, the crown may need to be removed before the symptoms will subside.

Recently crowned *anterior* teeth that exhibit percussion sensitivity can also be assessed in the same manner as a posterior tooth. If a single crown or fixed partial denture (bridge) has been made in an unduly upright position, it is difficult for the patient to move into a protrusive position without being obstructed. The patient may subject the tooth or teeth to abnormally high and potentially destructive occlusal forces in the protruded position during night clenching or grinding, resulting in pain. While adjustments are possible, replacement of the restorations may be necessary.

Other descriptions

Pain on swallowing

Pay particular attention to patients who may have undiagnosed pain on swallowing, particularly those who have not responded to antibiotics which may have been given on suspicion of a throat infection, and for whom no obvious cause is visible (e.g. swollen tonsils). The possibility of pharyngeal or laryngeal malignancy must be part of the differential diagnosis. Referral to an ENT specialist for examination is required. Lymph node involvement may be noticeable. Lymph node pathosis, stylohyoid calcifications and trigeminal neuralgia involving the glossopharyngeal or lingual nerve should be considered in a differential diagnosis and investigated. Patients with Eagle's syndrome (calcified stylohyoid ligament or elongated styloid process) can present with pain or discomfort on swallowing. The elongated process is visible radiographically. The pain on swallowing can be demonstrated by having the patient rotate the head to one side and move their jaw at the same time as swallowing.

Pain to tongue pressure

Patients may report that a tooth is sore to tongue pressure, sometimes after a restoration has been placed. *This tooth hurts when I press on it with my tongue.* The tongue is a powerful organ that contains eight distinct muscles. The pain the patient experiences simply may be due to the pressure from the tongue. Advising the patient *not to play with the tooth with their tongue* is sometimes the only treatment required. Similarly, patients who continually *check to see if a tooth is still sensitive* by grasping the tooth with a thumb and forefinger and wiggling it may be prolonging the pain or discomfort rather than just assessing its presence. These patients should be advised to discontinue the habit.

It is important to ascertain whether the pain is due to tongue movement, or whether the tooth is symptomatic because the tongue is pressing against the tooth. Although rare, patients may have trigeminal neuralgia involving the lingual nerve, which can be confused with tooth pain or pain produced by touching soft tissues.

Patients may report long-term discomfort in the intraoral soft tissues and constantly run their tongue over them. These patients may report this as tooth pain and demand treatment. A tongue or finger moving constantly over soft tissue can perpetuate sensitivity. Often an area on the attached gingiva can be identified which is red and shiny. A neuropathic origin is possible. In the absence of any obvious cause, the careful application of topical capsaicin cream can be used to desensitize the area.

Pain when traveling on an aircraft, diving or climbing

Orofacial pain can be initiated by a change in atmospheric pressure. The following terms are used when referring to the effects produced by these pressure changes:

- *Barodontalgia:* general term for pain that occurs due to changes in atmospheric pressure. It includes pain from an increase or decrease in pressure (e.g. the changes in pressure during flying, diving or climbing).
- *Aerodontalgia:* Pain in teeth that occurs when flying or climbing.
- *Barotrauma:* A general term used to describe tissue damage when atmospheric pressure increases.
- *Dental barotrauma:* A general term that describes damage and pain that occur in teeth as a result of increases in atmospheric pressure. It includes damage to restorations.
- *Barosinusitis:* Pain from the paranasal sinuses due to changes in atmospheric pressure.

Pain from barodontalgia can be severe and remain constant until atmospheric pressure returns to normal. Relief from aerodontalgia occurs during the descent of an aircraft from a high altitude. A diver gets relief from barodontalgia on return to the surface. It is easy to distinguish barosinusitis from barodontalgia, as barodontalgia is relieved when atmospheric pressure returns to normal.

The exact cause of barodontalgia has not been established, but stimulation of the nerve endings in an inflamed pulp or stimulation of nociceptors in the maxillary sinus with resultant pain referred to the teeth is thought to be responsible.[61] Most reported cases appear to be associated with teeth with pulpal pathosis. Acute or chronic periapical infections, caries, deep restorations, residual dental cysts, sinusitis, some cracked teeth and a history of recent surgery have been implicated.[62]

Useful questions to consider when suspecting pain from barodontalgia

For aerodontalgia:

Does the pain occur when the plane ascends or descends, or when it reaches a certain altitude?

Aerodontalgia is initiated when a plane ascends or has reached a certain altitude. It resolves when the aircraft descends. Barosinusitis, on the other hand, increases on descent.

For divers:

Does the pain occur when you are descending, at depth, or ascending to the surface?

Orofacial pain when diving that is initiated at depth and relieved during the ascent to the surface can be attributed to barodontalgia.

For both: *Does the pain continue once you return to the ground or the surface?*

Orofacial pain that lingers after the patient returns to normal atmospheric pressure can be attributed to barosinusitis.

Pain associated with exertion/pain after exertion

Cardiac pain (from angina) can be referred to the left mandible and very occasionally to the right. The pain may or may not radiate down the left arm.

Patients who report *aching* orofacial pain during or after physical exertion must be referred for immediate cardiac assessment, particularly if this pain occurs in the left mandible. There may be other associated signs and symptoms of cardiac disease, including breathlessness or ankle swelling. The possibility of referral of cardiac pain must also be considered if an ache in the left mandible cannot be attributed to any other cause. Orofacial pain that occurs during physical exertion can be sinus, neck, muscle or joint related, but this is usually associated with movement rather than exertion and does not develop as an ache.

Does the pain occur during or after physical exertion and does it go away immediately after you stop?

Cardiac disease may cause an *aching* pain in the left mandible during or after exertion.

Chapter 9

Analyzing Pain Descriptions – Time Analysis and the Diagnosis of Orofacial Pain

Alex J. Moule and M. Lamar Hicks

"When did the pain start?"
"Where did the pain start?"

Introduction

Assessing time-related pain characteristics is important when developing a differential diagnosis for a patient with orofacial pain. Recognizing that most painful conditions follow distinct time-related patterns makes diagnosis easier. Although dental pain can mimic many other conditions, in its acute phase this commonest cause of orofacial pain follows a distinct and identifiable time-related pattern. The question *"When did the pain start?"* is nevertheless only one of the time-related questions. Depending on the complexity of the case and what information a patient volunteers, answers to some or many of the following questions may also be required:

- *"Are you in pain now?"*
- *"When did the pain start?"*
- *"When does the pain start?"*
- *"How often does the pain occur?"*
- *"How long does the pain last?"*
- *"How long have you been experiencing the pain you have right now?"*
- *"When do you get the pain?"*
- *"Has the pain changed over time?"*
- *"How has the pain changed over time?"*
- *"Does the pain change during the day?"*
- *"Do you feel the pain follows any pattern?"*
- *"Have you had this pain before?"*
- *"When did you have this pain before?"*
- *"How often have you had this pain before?"*

None of these questions by themselves are diagnostic, and not all of them are required for simple cases. However, answers to specific questioning form an important framework for a diagnostic continuum that develops observable patterns. These patterns assist the diagnostician to formulate a differential diagnosis, the individual components of which can be assessed, ruled out or confirmed by screening.

If we remember the complexity of pain pathways, and that pain from irreversible pulpitis or muscle dysfunction can be referred from one location to a more distant site, the question *"Where did the pain start?"* becomes an important part of time-related questioning. *The location where the pain started is likely to identify the source of pain.* Even though a patient's interpretation of events is not always accurate, also asking the question *"What do you think started this pain?"* helps to define a timeline.

The duration and other characteristics of pain are influenced by measures that patients or practitioners take to relieve the pain and by certain factors that prolong it. Thus, time-related questioning goes hand-in-hand with the positive and negative factors that influence the chief complaint. Investigating and elucidating these factors are part of the strategy for selecting general screening questions presented earlier in this manual:

- *"Does anything make the pain worse"*
- *"Does anything make the pain better?"*
- *"Does medication help to relieve the pain?"*

This chapter discusses the relevance of time-related questioning in establishing a differential diagnosis for patients with orofacial pain.

Diagnosing Dental and Orofacial Pain: A Clinical Manual, First Edition. Edited by Alex J. Moule and M. Lamar Hicks.
© 2017 John Wiley & Sons, Ltd. Published 2017 by John Wiley & Sons, Ltd.
Companion website: www.wiley.com/go/moule/dental_and_orofacial_pain

Are you in pain now?

Many orofacial pain problems are easier to diagnose if the patient is examined when the pain is present at the time of examination. This is especially true with recurrent or intermittent pain where a diagnosis is suspected, but where the signs and symptoms are not present. For example, cluster headache and angioneurotic edema, two dissimilar conditions, are much easier to diagnose if the patient has the signs and/or symptoms at the time of examination. If the diagnosis is uncertain, it may be made clearer by asking the patient to return, if possible, when the pain is present. A photograph taken on a mobile phone is useful for communicating information immediately to a practitioner.

Many patients in pain come to your office having taken substantial doses of analgesic medications, which complicates assessment and makes testing difficult. Patients may have to return for diagnosis later when the analgesic effects have worn off. For the protection of both the patient and the clinician, those patients who appear to be under the influence of medication, drugs or alcohol, and do not need emergency relief of pain, should be reappointed or referred for specialist care.

When did the pain start?

The starting point for the patient's pain is important as it establishes the beginning of a definitive timeline, which broadly separates acute pain from chronic pain. Patients may volunteer the information that there is an association between the commencement of the pain and a certain event or treatment. This information, combined with how the pain has changed over time, facilitates a process of broad sorting. Unfortunately, an individual's recollection of events and interpretation of cause may not always be accurate, and this information must be corroborated.

When does the pain start?

Pain can be spontaneous or initiated by an event or a stimulus. If pain is initiated by hot or cold liquids, a dental cause is invariably present (see Chapter 12). Identification of stimulating factors and any association with specific activities should be noted in descriptions of daily patterns.

How often does the pain occur?
How long does the pain last?

These two questions, when *used together*, help to establish a time-defined pain pattern. How often the pain occurs and how long it lasts should be recorded diagrammatically in seconds, minutes, hours or days, as can the severity of the pain, severity being indicated by lines and time in words (see Chapter 5, Figs 5-1 to 5-5). Most painful orofacial conditions follow a time-related pattern that is distinctive. Analgesic medications and other palliative measures taken to prevent or relieve the pain are confounding factors.

A short stab of pain that recurs during the day and only lasts for a few seconds (e.g. trigeminal neuralgia) paints a different picture from a pain that ebbs and flows over many hours (e.g. irreversible pulpitis), or one that lasts for weeks (e.g. muscle pain). Acute pain usually remains at a constant level or increases in intensity until treatment or a natural compensatory change occurs (e.g. surgically induced or spontaneous drainage of an acute abscess). Chronic pain, which can last months or years, on the other hand, can vary in its expression and can be dependent on daily activity and life events. The acute pain of migraine and cluster headache usually lasts for only a few hours. Tension headaches can last for days. Muscle pain can last for months.

How long have you been experiencing the pain you have right now?

This question is more specific from the above and obtains information on the actual presenting pain profile, although the information obtained may be similar. Severe dental pain usually lasts for only a few days. Of diagnostic importance, therefore, is that the longer a pain has been present, the less likely there is a dental origin. Anecdotally, the larger the pulp in a tooth with pulpitis the longer the pain will be present. Thus, for example, a molar tooth with a large pulp is more likely to be the cause of longer term acute pulpitis than an adjacent molar tooth with a calcified pulp chamber.

Patients with current *long-term pain* require special management. Chronic pain is variously described in the literature as lasting more than 3 to 6 months. Although some patients can be helped by treatment (e.g. those with cervicogenic headaches due to whiplash injuries), many patients need long-term medication, psychological support and specialized help with pain management. The close relationship between chronic pain and a multitude of interrelated psychosocial factors cannot be overemphasized. If no obvious problem can be found for a patient with chronic pain, referral for diagnosis and management by a pain specialist is recommended (see Chapter 23).

Care should be taken to avoid invasive treatment for a patient with chronic pain, unless a specific diagnosis has been made and a need for treatment is clearly established. Intervention without conclusive evidence, even when a patient fervently insists that treatment be performed, is rarely in the best interest of the patient or the practitioner.

When do you get the pain?
Does the pain change during the day?

This broad line of questioning is similar to "*When does the pain start?*" It is, however, more encompassing. It allows patients to explain where they are and what they are doing when the pain commences, and at what time of day it occurs. The information of *when and where does it happen,* when taken together, can be diagnostically important. An assessment of the repetition and regularity of changes in pain experience (e.g. three times a day, once a day, or four or five times in a week) is necessary. Although there are numerous possibilities, a number of broad generalizations are possible.

As discussed previously, each time a patient responds to a question, the response requires assessment: *What does that answer mean? What more do I need to know?* Most pain associations are easy to interpret if considered separately (e.g. in the afternoon, when I go out in the cold, or when I lie down, sit up or bend down). *Pain that has a regular daily pattern is unlikely to be dental pain.* Thus, if patients describe time-related occurrences (at work, on the weekend, 4:00 am, mid-morning, in the middle of the afternoon or late at night), they are not describing dental pain.

Similarly, and importantly, the intensity of pulpal pain does not remain constant, but changes over time. The character and intensity of the pain ebb and flow. Sometimes the pain becomes intense and unbearable; other times it is no more than a background discomfort. Orofacial pain that is constant in intensity is again unlikely to be dental, and is often of muscle origin. Inflammation of the maxillary sinus that involves the ostium can cause a constant ache that can last for hours (see Chapter 16, Figs 16-2 and 16-3).

Chronic orofacial pain can increase or decrease in intensity, depending on the patient's functional, work-related or social activities during the day. Pain that intensifies during the day is different from a pain that gets better during the day. A pain that has a distinct pattern and duration (e.g. migraine) is distinct from one that may occur randomly throughout the day (e.g. pulpitis). Analyzing these associations (where and what) allows broad generalizations to be made when patients describe time-related pain. This in turn allows appropriate screening to take place.

Pain that occurs at a specific time each day

Special emphasis should be placed on a patient's response if an exact time of day is stipulated (e.g. "Four o'clock in the morning" or "3:00 pm".). In these circumstances, record the pattern and screen initially for cluster headache.

Pain on waking in the morning

Any pain that has a daily pattern is highly unlikely to be of *dental* origin. Orofacial pain presenting in the morning is commonly muscle related due to night-time clenching or night-time bruxism. Patients who have headaches upon waking may have cervicogenic problems. Referral to a physiotherapist is often helpful. Patients can also awake in the morning with a cluster headache. Of note is that many patients with chronic orofacial pain report poor sleep patterns.[63] When considering *morning pain*, some important questions to consider are:

Does the pain wake them up?
Screen initially for pulpitis, cluster headaches and night-time clenching.
Is the pain present when they wake up?
Screen for sinusitis, muscle pain or a rare intracranial lesion.
Does the pain only occur after they wake up? (e.g. once they start talking or eating)
Screen for trigeminal neuralgia.
Does the pain get better when they get up?
Screen for chronic sinusitis and muscle dysfunction.
Does the pain develop during the morning?
Screen for daytime clenching, occupational and environmental factors, and chronic sinusitis.

Pain in the afternoon or evening

Pain that occurs in the afternoon or evening is usually of muscle origin and associated with stress or daytime bruxism. People who work long hours on *computers* in uncomfortable positions, or operate a *computer mouse* in an awkward position, frequently develop neck or orofacial pain that worsens as the day progresses. Similarly, office workers who hold a phone between their shoulder and lower jaw may develop neck or orofacial pain. Musicians can also develop neck, joint and muscle discomfort. In the absence of a cluster headache (which has specific time characteristics), patients who develop pain as the day progresses should be screened for occupational and environmental causes. Patients with trigeminal neuropathic orofacial pain can also have a daily pattern to their pain experience, the intensity of which may vary according to daily activities and life events.

How has the pain changed over time?
Is there any pattern to how it changes?
Establishing how the pain behaves over time is valuable from both diagnostic and treatment perspectives. If there is no obvious pathological problem that needs urgent treatment, orofacial pain that is manageable and that *may be getting better* should be left untreated. The patient should be periodically recalled for evaluation. Treatment interventions should be avoided due to the risk that associated local reactions to this may complicate the diagnostic process. This is often the case with patients with undiagnosed chronic facial pain, where treatment can exacerbate or create new symptoms.

Pain that is increasing in severity requires expeditious diagnosis and urgent treatment. Be wary of a patient who reports severe pain and demands treatment and/or medication where the signs and symptoms do not match the reported pain profile.[63] The possibility of drug dependence must be considered.

Be wary also if a patient seeks treatment for a first-time headache that is increasing in severity for which no obvious cause can be established. The possibility of a carotid dissection or intracranial lesion has to be considered.[64]

Have you had the pain before?
When did you have this pain before?
How often have you had this pain before?

Patients may not volunteer information of a history of orofacial pain, and may relate this information only when specifically asked. The above series of cascading questions establishes past experience. Patients who respond positively should be questioned as to whether they feel that their present pain is the *same pain as before*. Details of the patient's history, including the treatment that was provided and whether the treatment was successful, should be carefully considered when assessing difficult-to-diagnose orofacial pain problems that do not add up to a diagnosis of pulpal pain. Take care not to rely completely on a patient's recall of past events. A final and definitive diagnosis must be confirmed before any treatment is performed.

In summary, most orofacial pain problems follow a distinct time-related pattern. Assessing these characteristics is important when developing a differential diagnosis. Responses help to establish a pattern. Not all of the above time-related questions are necessary to establish a diagnosis. Rather, they are screening questions where responses direct a second line of specific questioning and/or testing. Questioning is continued if a diagnosis is not apparent. Detail required is dependent on the complexity of the case.

Chapter 10

Analyzing Pain Descriptions – Factors Influencing the Pain

Alex J. Moule and M. Lamar Hicks

Relief of pain

The manner in which a patient has been able to gain pain relief is significant. This chapter concentrates on how reactions to past medications and other therapies can be used as diagnostic tools in assessing a patient's current problems. A patient's response to specific medication (e.g. carbamazepine if trigeminal neuralgia is suspected, or diazepam if muscle spasm or tension headache is suspected) can confirm that a "probable" diagnosis is correct. Other associations that are diagnostically significant are how maxillary sinusitis responds to decongestant medication or steam inhalation, how joint pain responds to non-steroidal anti-inflammatory medication and how massage or physical therapy relieves muscle pain or cervicogenic headache. Responses to heat and cold are covered in Chapter 9.

Analgesics and pain diagnosis

An assessment of a patient's response to analgesic medication may suggest the type of orofacial pain the patient is experiencing. Questioning should include:

"Does anything make the pain worse?"
"Does anything make the pain better?"
"Does medication help to relieve the pain?"

Most dental pain can be controlled effectively by regular analgesics such as paracetamol (acetaminophen), codeine or ibuprofen (Fig. 10-1). The likelihood of a non-dental cause increases if the orofacial pain is not controlled or eliminated with these drugs used singly, in combination or in staggered doses. Muscle and joint pains usually do not respond well to paracetamol, but do well to moist heat and medications containing muscle relaxants. If a patient obtains relief from these medications (e.g. diazepam) they should be screened for psychosomatic and non-odontogenic pain, including muscle pain.

Pay attention to patients who describe the severity of pain by the number of analgesic pills they have taken. An example is a patient who states that *"This was a six-Panadol headache!"* These patients may be overmedicating or attention seeking. Patients may demand a prescription for strong pain medications, including narcotics, to relieve the pain. If the condition they are describing does not fit the pain that appears to be present, or if they demand a particular medication, the probability that these patients are drug seekers is very high. Drug dependency must be considered. Referral of the patient or a telephone call to their general medical practitioner is appropriate. Many seemingly normal patients can be addicted to over-the-counter analgesics, muscle relaxants or other prescription medications. A suspicion of this dependence is raised when the patient's pain does not appear to be interfering with sleep or daily function.

Pay attention to patients who arrive for pain diagnosis with a history of prescriptions for a large number of analgesic medications. Although patients may have been prescribed drugs by a variety of well-meaning practitioners, compliance with treatment instructions should be questioned. This is especially true if a patient presents for diagnosis with a bag of medication or a detailed list of medications they have tried. Some questions to ask are:

"Are you taking anything for the pain?"
"How many pain pills are you taking?"
"Is this helping to control the pain?"
"Did you complete the prescribed course of treatment?"

Diagnosing Dental and Orofacial Pain: A Clinical Manual, First Edition. Edited by Alex J. Moule and M. Lamar Hicks.
© 2017 John Wiley & Sons, Ltd. Published 2017 by John Wiley & Sons, Ltd.
Companion website: www.wiley.com/go/moule/dental_and_orofacial_pain

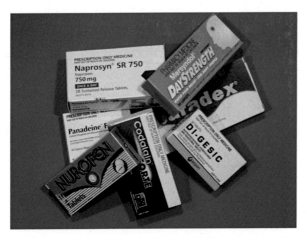

Fig. 10-1 Most dental pain can be controlled to some extent by regular analgesics. Patients who do not obtain relief and who do not have obvious signs of dental pathology may not be suffering pain of dental origin.

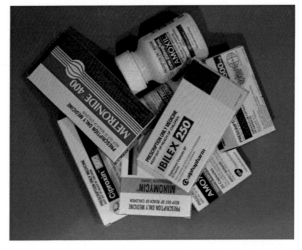

Fig. 10-2 A patient's response to recently prescribed antibiotics can assist in determining the cause of their discomfort.

Local anaesthesia and pain diagnosis

If local anaesthesia does not relieve the pain, it is highly unlikely that pain is of dental origin. Similarly if a patient reports only short-term relief (only minutes from local analgesia), it is also unlikely that there is a dental origin to the pain. The patient may be suffering from neuropathic orofacial pain.

Selective anesthesia involves anesthetizing selective areas or regions. The role of selective anesthesia in pain diagnosis is discussed in Chapter 11. Selectively anesthetizing a tooth, several teeth or an arch can be helpful in identifying a painful tooth. If pain is relieved with anesthesia, then the source of the pain is within the anesthetized area. Selective anesthesia is particularly useful if there is confusion regarding the arch in which the sensitive tooth is located, in excluding certain teeth as the source of pain, or in confirming that pain is or is not arising from a particular site; for example, pain of muscle origin is not relieved by local anesthesia unless the anesthetic solution is injected into the muscle trigger points.[65]

Antibiotics and pain diagnosis

The over-prescription of antibiotics for the treatment of dental and orofacial pain problems is well known. Thus, many patients arrive for diagnosis with a history of taking antibiotic medication (Fig. 10-2). Assessing a patient's reaction to this medication can provide information on the current problem.

In the absence of a definitive dental diagnosis, a patient's response to recently prescribed antibiotic medication has to be taken into consideration. This can be helpful in determining whether an infective cause is present. If antibiotics provided pain relief, an infection may be the cause. However, care should be taken in interpreting the patient's response to antibiotics. *Time must also be taken into consideration.* Most dental infections respond well to antibiotic medication, usually within 48 to 72 hours. Thus, if a patient

received antibiotics and the pain improved within this time period, the problem was most likely caused by infection. If there is no improvement at all, a dental cause is not eliminated, as patients with irreversible pulpitis do not respond to antibiotics, but a dental infection or other infection is less likely. If the improvement took longer than a few days (e.g. a whole week, or "needed two courses of antibiotics"), it is possible that the pain resolved due to the *passage of time* rather than as a result of antibiotic medication.

A common scenario is a patient who reports pain under the jaw and is regularly prescribed antibiotics because *"my glands are up again"*. These patients may take more than a week to get better and may even require *"a second course of antibiotics"*. Invariably patients are reporting pain in the suprahyoid muscles, likely the posterior belly of the digastric muscle, and that is being misinterpreted as *swollen glands*. This pain usually resolves over time without antibiotics. These patients should be screened for TMD and, if necessary, referred for physical therapy.

There are other situations where patient responses are illogical and an infection is definitely not involved. An example is the patient who states, *"I took one or two antibiotic tablets and the pain went away."* In these cases, the antibiotic has had nothing to do with the resolution of the pain. It is probable that the placebo effect is responsible for the patient's dramatic recovery. Thus, screening questions that need to be asked together are:

"Have you been on antibiotics?"
"Did the antibiotics help with the pain?"
"How long have the antibiotics taken to work?"

Endodontics and pain diagnosis

Patients often present for pain diagnosis who have had endodontic procedures and who are still experiencing pain. The patient may be concerned that the endodontic treatment should be redone or even that endodontic surgery may be needed. Alternatively, practitioners may keep replacing intra-canal dressings in the hope that the discomfort will resolve. Before any further treatment is undertaken, three related questions need to be asked:

"Did the root canal treatment make any difference to the pain you were having?"

If the current endodontic treatment has not changed the character of the pain, then a pulpal problem was not the cause of pain. Further endodontic management to treat the pain is not warranted. This is especially true if the pulp was vital at the time it was extirpated (removed). Except in the case of acute dental infections, endodontic treatment should quickly change the character of the presenting pain. If there was a *pulpal problem*, removal of the pulp should immediately relieve the pain or change the character of the pain. Therefore, look elsewhere.

"Is the pain you are having right now the same type of pain you were having before treatment?"

This question is similar to the first question, but very important when dealing with patients with chronic orofacial pain who have had extensive treatment and are still in pain. Sometimes these patients insist that a particular treatment procedure be redone and/or may be critical of the quality of work that has been performed. If the quality and character of the pain have not changed over time, redoing work will not help the patient. The problem is unrelated to any treatment performed. A similar scenario involves a patient who reports suffering exactly the *same pain as they had originally* after the dental anesthesia used during treatment has worn off. Before further treatment, a definitive diagnosis needs to be established.

NOTE: If endodontic management relieves the pain, it can be assumed that the pulp was the source of the discomfort.

If endodontic management has not relieved a patient's discomfort, then an alternative cause of this discomfort must be established. Redoing treatment procedures will not relieve the pain.

Did the dentist have any trouble numbing up the tooth?

If the tooth was hard to anesthetize, *the pulp was vital*. If the patient was still in pain after the pulp was removed, the pain was not related to this tooth. Extraction or further endodontic management will not alleviate the pain, nor will endodontic management on an adjoining tooth, particularly on the contralateral side. Anecdotally, patients suffering trigeminal neuropathic orofacial pain (including atypical odontalgia) regularly report that their tooth was very *hard to numb up* before the pulp was removed, or that the endodontic treatment was extremely painful.

If a situation like this *does not add up* and there are red-flag warning signs of a non-odontogenic cause for a toothache, early referral for diagnosis is advised before any treatment is undertaken (see Chapter 22). *The best place for a patient can be in someone else's office.*

CAUTION: Take particular care when diagnosing pain in a patient who presents with a painful anterior tooth under going endodontic treatment and who reports that the dentist had trouble numbing the tooth up to remove the pulp. If the tooth was difficult to anesthetize, then the pulp was vital when it was treated. A non-odontogenic cause has to be suspected if there is continuance of pain, particularly the *same* pain.

Thus a patient's reaction to local analgesia, analgesics, antibiotic therapy and any treatment procedures must be analyzed carefully in the presence of any continuing pain. *If the treatment modifies or relieves the pain, then it is likely there is an association with the procedure and the painful state.* If there is no demonstrable symptomic relief or change in the quality and severity of the original pain, it is unlikely that redoing the procedure will have an effect on symptoms or that the tooth under treatment is the cause of the discomfort.

Chapter 11

Tests and Testing

Alex J. Moule and Unni Krishnan

Pulp sensibility (vitality) tests

A common misconception of clinicians when encountering a patient in pain is the perceived necessity to perform a battery of thermal and electrical pulp tests on multiple teeth to determine the state of the pulp. This pulp sensibility testing is usually carried out by observing the response of teeth to a thermal or electrical stimulus. A cold stimulus is applied using carbon dioxide (CO_2) snow (–56 to –98 °C), refrigerant sprays (e.g. Endo-ice®) (–26 °C) or ice. CO_2 snow and refrigerant sprays provide more predictable responses than ice, particularly for crowned teeth.[66]

The intensity of the response to the stimulus and the continuance of pain after stimulation are used as measures of the health of the pulp. Calcified teeth or teeth with pulp canal obliteration will have a yellowish discoloration and usually will not respond to thermal testing (Fig. 11-1). This is due to the larger bulk of coronal dentin which prevents the transfer of the thermal stimulus to the pulp. Pulps in calcified canals usually respond to electrical stimulation (Fig. 11-2).

Pulp testing, however, does not always accurately determine the status of the pulp.[67] *In many cases, it is determined from the history and not from testing.* With dental pain diagnosis, the task for the clinician is often not to determine the state of the pulp, but rather to determine the *identity of the aching tooth.* Pulp testing procedures are of most value:

- when the tooth is expected to be vital.
- in trauma situations where sensibility testing is necessary to establish a baseline for later reference.
- for exclusion in situations where the identity of a non-responsive tooth is important and the response of adjacent teeth must be assessed (dental infections).

- for ensuring that all teeth are responsive in difficult diagnostic situations where pain of non-odontogenic origin is suspected.
- in a pre-operative assessment of pulpal status before planning restorations.

Pulp testing may not be useful in determining the identity of an aching tooth. There is little value in assessing the vitality of every tooth in an arch if the patient is complaining of sensitivity to thermal changes.

There is a *BIG* difference between tooth identification and pulp sensibility testing. Recognizing the difference between the two is important. The identification of a painful tooth is much easier if there are associated periradicular symptoms. Nine out of 10 patients can identify a painful tooth if periradicular symptoms are present, whereas less than one-third of emergency dental patients are capable of correctly locating the offending tooth in the absence of these.[68] This may be due to the limited number of proprioceptive (localization) nerve fibers in the pulp, which prevents localization of the offending tooth when inflammation is limited only to the pulp.[69] In addition, a wider two-point discrimination seems to exist in posterior teeth. Hence, there is more difficulty for a patient to accurately identify a painful posterior tooth as compared to an anterior tooth.[68,70] Identification is further complicated by pain being referred 25% of the time to the opposing arch or too an adjacent tooth 80% of the time.[71]

NOTE: Pain from a pulpitis does not cross the midline unless the source is in the midline.

For tooth identification, it is better to reproduce the patient's pain (chief complaint) under the conditions that cause the tooth to be painful. Thus, if there

Diagnosing Dental and Orofacial Pain: A Clinical Manual, First Edition. Edited by Alex J. Moule and M. Lamar Hicks.
© 2017 John Wiley & Sons, Ltd. Published 2017 by John Wiley & Sons, Ltd.
Companion website: www.wiley.com/go/moule/dental_and_orofacial_pain

(A)

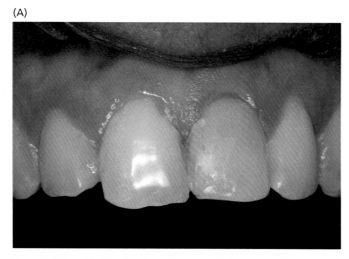

(B)

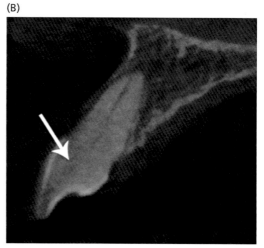

Fig. 11-1 Yellowish discoloration of maxillary left central incisor suggestive of pulp canal obliteration (calcific metamorphosis) (A). Sagittal cone beam computed tomography (CBCT) image of the maxillary left central (B) incisor shows calcification of the coronal pulp (arrow).

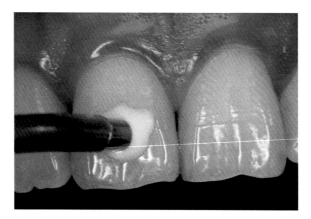

Fig. 11-2 An electric pulp test is also a useful means of assessing the sensibility of a pulp in a tooth, particularly when the pulps are calcified. Calcified teeth often do not respond to cold testing due to the bulk of dentin between the stimulus and the pulp.

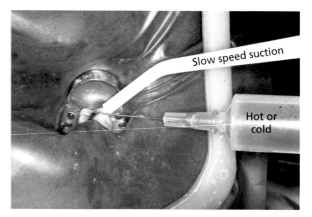

Fig. 11-3 Bathing individual teeth in hot or cold water under rubber dam isolation will quickly disclose the identity of a temperature-sensitive tooth. Each tooth is isolated individually and bathed for a few seconds. Where a delayed response to heat is reported, the teeth should be bathed in hot water, with adequate time to react to this stimulus, before the next tooth is tested.

is pain from biting only, then use a bite test. If the patient reports that the tooth is painful to cold, use cold water for testing (water bath test). If the tooth is painful to heat, use hot water for testing. If the tooth is sensitive to sweetness, test it with a sweet solution.

If a history of temperature sensitivity is elicited, tooth identification is relatively easy. Testing teeth individually with hot or cold water under rubber dam isolation will very quickly disclose the identity of the temperature-sensitive tooth (Fig. 11-3). Some teeth with pulpitis can be sensitive to heat, but their pain can be relieved by the application of cold. Thus, unless the patient reports extreme sensitivity to cold, identification may more reliably be made using *hot water*. Indeed, some patients with severely symptomatic irreversible pulpitis come to the dental office carrying ice or very cold water, which they use for pain relief. When using hot or cold water to identify aching teeth:

- Isolate the teeth individually.
- Test the teeth systematically.

- Be thorough and test all teeth in a quadrant or arch.
- As water can pool posteriorly, test the most posterior teeth first.
- If testing with hot water, do not use the high-speed evacuator until the patient is given time to respond to the stimulus, as this can have a cooling effect.

The literature suggests the need to compare the response of one tooth with another using a cold testing device, such as CO_2 snow or refrigerant sprays (Fig. 11-4). While this may be useful in some circumstances, the actual condition of pulp cannot be determined by this comparative testing.[67] Indeed, for pulp testing, *any level of response is a "response" and is a probable indicator for pulp vitality*. However, as far as tooth identification is concerned, the responses that are the most diagnostic are those which are *severe, prolonged exacerbate the patient's pain*, or, in the case of a suspected non-vital tooth (tooth with a necrotic pulp), are negative.

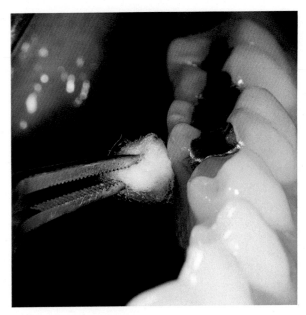

Fig. 11-4 Testing the lingual surface of mandibular molars often gives a more reliable testing result.

While it is uncommon for teeth to give a response to pulp testing and also to be associated with dental infection, this possibility has to be considered. Vital inflamed pulp tissue can exist apically in some teeth, even in the presence of periradicular radiolucency.[72] Furthermore, despite the presence of an apparently avascular pulp, sensory nerves (c-fibers) can remain functional in the apical portion of the pulp canal, reacting to heat, as neural tissues are generally more resistant to breakdown from inflammatory processes.[73]

NOTE: In most mandibular molar teeth, sensibility testing is usually more predictable if the occlusal third of the lingual surfaces are tested, rather than the buccal surface, especially if restorations are present. In mandibular molar teeth, the dentin overlying the pulp is usually thinner here than the buccal dentin.

All teeth with periapical radiolucencies must be tested for pulp sensibility in order to exclude other more sinister causes, including tumors or lesions not involving the pulp, or periapical bone loss.

NOTE: When interpreting results of pulp testing, remember that 80 to 85% of patients with moderate to severe pain may have taken analgesics.[74] This can significantly alter the response of the patient to palpation, percussion and pulp sensibility tests and make diagnosis more difficult.[75]

Percussion

Percussion testing is useful for the identification of many painful teeth. In almost all cases percussion testing should be done in comparison with adjacent teeth. The patient is asked to compare the response on several teeth rather than testing just a single tooth. The suspected tooth should not be tested first, and all teeth should be tested in a random order. In cases where there is extreme sensitivity, care should be taken of course to avoid percussing immediately with an instrument, but rather start first by gently touching the tooth with a finger.

STATE: *I am going to tap on these teeth. Call this one number one, call this one number two, and call this one number three. Which one was more sensitive to the tapping?* If a patient reports a particular tooth may be more sensitive than another, then test again in a different order for confirmation (Fig. 11-5).

Except in the case of overt infection (e.g. an abscess), be wary if a patient reports that more than one tooth is sensitive to percussion, or where percussion testing is inconsistent. In the absence of alveolar fracture or overt infection, a non-dental cause for the chief complaint, such as clenching, maxillary sinusitis or trigeminal neuropathic orofacial pain, must be considered.

Experimental studies have shown that percussion sensitivity can be measured in endodontic patients using bite force transducers.[76] Although not yet currently practical or cost-effective for routine diagnostic use, this technology may prove useful in diagnosis, particularly in patients with irreversible pulpitis and who have taken analgesics.[75]

Palpation

Palpation of both intra-oral and extra-oral tissues should always be carried out when examining a patient who has a chief complaint of pain. The location of a painful swelling or area of tenderness in relation to the root apex is important. Tenderness is usually apically located in teeth with periapical pathosis. With periodontal lesions (e.g. periodontal abscesses and vertical root fractures), tenderness is more likely elicited in the mid-root region or gingivally.

There are occasions when root apices fenestrate the buccal bone. Careful palpation of the bony housing around these teeth should enable an astute clinician to detect apical root fenestrations, especially around the buccal roots of maxillary premolars or molars and some maxillary anterior teeth (Fig. 11-8). These teeth can present with apical sensitivity, but with no apparent periapical radiolucency, as the pathosis is not confined within the bone. Cases where root apices fenestrate the bony housing have been associated with persistent pain after root canal treatment, even in teeth that appear radiographically to have optimal root canal fillings.[77] Cone beam computed tomography (CBCT) is often required to confirm the diagnosis (Fig. 11-6).

Periodontal probing

Routine periodontal probing must be carried out as part of pain diagnosis (Fig. 11-7). The differences in bone loss patterns and periodontal probing defects due to periodontal disease and those found with

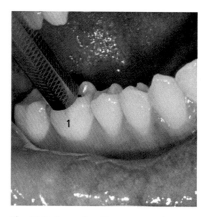
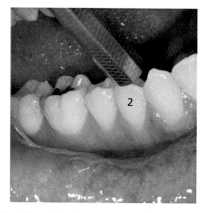
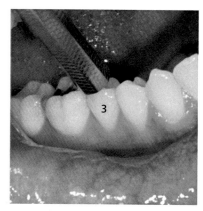

Fig. 11-5 Assessing the response to percussion. Determine the comparative response to a percussive blow on adjacent teeth. Once a response has been observed, retest the teeth in a different order to confirm the identity of the percussion-sensitive tooth.

(A)   (B)

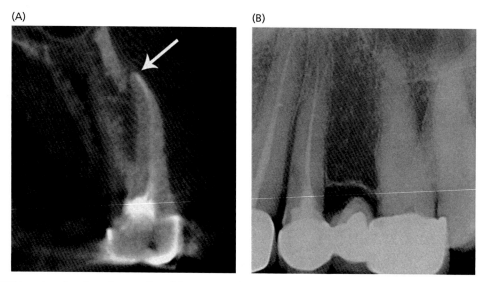

Fig. 11-6 CBCT imaging showing a fenestration of the root apex (arrowed) in an endodontically treated first premolar tooth with sensitivity to palpation over the buccal cortex near the root apex (A). The fenestration is not visible on the periapical radiograph (B). Radiographic changes are not apparent on the periapical radiograph as the inflammatory reaction is external to the confines of the surrounding bone.

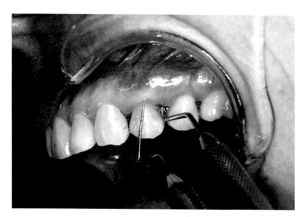

Fig. 11-7 A maxillary first premolar tooth with an isolated deep probing pocket on the distal marginal ridge in an otherwise healthy periodontium. This is an indication that a vertical root fracture is present. Note normal probing depth on the buccal.

vertical root fractures are important to distinguish. In periodontal disease the probing defect is often wide and deep and can involve multiple teeth, whereas in a vertical root fracture the defect is consistently narrower, deep and isolated to a single tooth. The deep probing defect may be unilateral or bilateral.[78]

Radiographs

The radiographic examination required for pain diagnosis is dependent on the presenting pathology and the degree of difficulty in diagnosing the patient's pain. With a temperature-sensitive tooth with reversible pulpitis, a standard bitewing radiograph may be all that is necessary. A well-oriented periapical radiograph is, however, essential when examining teeth with irreversible pulpitis, or teeth showing signs or symptoms of periodontal or periapical disease.

NOTE: Periapical changes may not be immediately evident after a pulp becomes necrotic. Thus, if difficulty is experienced in identifying a painful tooth, or if a tooth exhibits periapical pain, do not accept a radiograph that is more than a few days old.

While a straight-on periapical view is usually the most useful, a tube shift or altered-angle image can be useful in identifying trifurcation bone loss in upper molars, and in separating roots and root apices from superimposed anatomical structures:

- Do not accept a radiograph that is underdeveloped, underexposed or not correctly oriented.
- Do not accept a radiograph where the root apex is not in the center of the film.
- If an unusual structure is present on a periapical film, confirm this observation with a second radiograph before trying to diagnose it.
- Do not accept a film where the entire periphery of the lesion cannot be seen.
- If the entire lesion is not completely visible on the radiograph, identify why the error was made before taking another film or getting a larger view.

A panoramic image (OPG) (Fig. 11-8) is a useful screening radiograph for the more difficult cases. This provides a good overview of the TM joints, complete dentition and upper and lower jaws. If a sinusitis is present, it can also show cloudiness in the maxillary sinuses. CT scans are the images of choice to determine sinus *disease*. However, imaging only shows the pathology that is present at the time the image was taken. A radiographic image of a sinus taken a few days after an infection may show little evidence of the pathologic condition. Not all sinus infections are visible radiographically.

Cone beam computed tomography

Considering the additional radiation associated with CBCT, its use should be limited to elusive cases of orofacial pain. Clinical examination and meticulous history taking remain the critical steps in diagnosing orofacial pain. CBCT does, however, have a role to play in hard-to-diagnose cases with poorly localized signs and symptoms (Figs 11-9 and 11-10). Studies have shown that 17% of cases previously categorized as having *atypical odontalgia* (non-dental causes of orofacial pain – see Chapter 3) had periapical bone

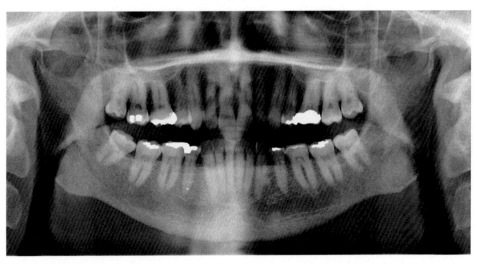

Fig. 11-8 An OPG is a good screening radiograph. It provides a good overview of the dentition, the supporting structures and the temporomandibular joints.

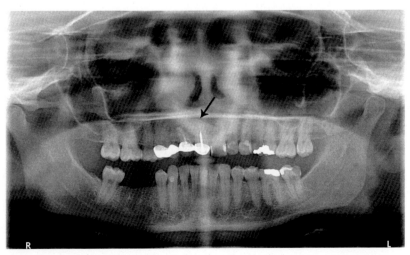

Fig. 11-9 OPG of a 37-year-old male complaining of persistent pain in his upper central incisor region. Note the lack of definition of the periapical regions of the maxillary and mandibular anterior teeth in OPG due to superimposition of other anatomic structures and the presence of an impacted maxillary canine (arrow), but the cause of the discomfort is not obvious. This became apparent with CBCT imaging (Fig. 11-10).

(A)   (B)   (C)

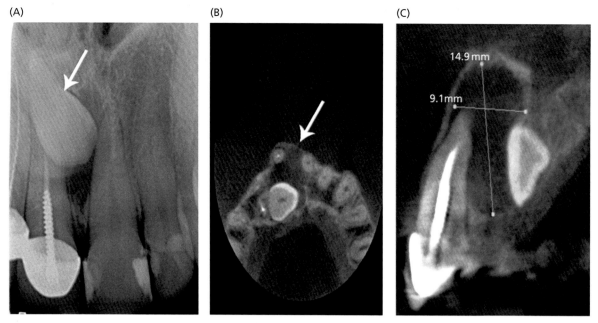

Fig. 11-10 An example how CBCT imaging can assist with diagnosis and show the full extent of a lesion.

destruction when CBCT was used as a diagnostic tool.[79] Similar studies report that CBCT is more accurate in diagnosing periapical pathosis, identifying nearly 20% more periapical lesions than periapical radiographs in non-endodontically treated teeth with necrotic pulps.[80]

(a) A periapical radiograph confirmed the presence of an impacted tooth with a coronal midline radiolucency and endodontically treated maxillary right central incisor. The left central incisor has responded normally to pulp sensibility tests. Based on these findings, differential diagnosis of endodontic pathosis, pathology associated with impacted tooth or infected nasopalatine cyst was made.

(b) Axial CBCT slices revealed asymmetrical expansion of the lesion excluding a nasopalatine cyst and no circumferential radiolucency associated with the crown of the impacted maxillary canine. The radiolucency was associated with a right maxillary central incisor (arrows), with expansion and perforation of labial cortex.

(c) Sagittal slices confirmed the relationship of the lesion with the inadequate endodontic treatment on the maxillary right central incisor.

Bite testing

Pain on biting has to be distinguished from pain on percussion (see Chapter 8). Some teeth that respond painfully to biting forces are not painful to percussive blows. A prime example of this is a cracked tooth, where a tooth can be sensitive to biting pressure, but may not be to percussion. With a cracked tooth, pain on percussion is often elicited only if the percussive blow is in a direction that activates the crack. Similarly, pain arising from occlusal interferences,

particularly where the tooth is only in traumatic occlusion for a small part of an excursive movement, may not be reproduced by a percussion test.

Several proprietary products are available for bite testing, for example Fracfinder® (www.denbur.com) and Tooth Slooth® (www.toothslooth.com) (Fig. 11-11). While these products are useful in identifying the location of a bite-sensitive tooth or cusp, with difficult-to-diagnose cracked teeth they are not always useful because:

- It is not always possible to exert sufficient pressure on non-working cusps.
- The maximum biting force occurs when teeth are almost in contact, rather than when they are separated by a few millimetres.

Whatever device is used to test responses to biting in difficult-to-diagnose cracked teeth, it should be

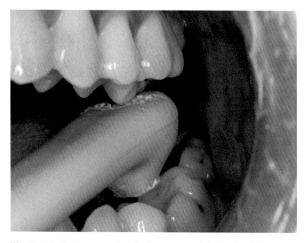

Fig. 11-11 Systematically placing a propriety device between the teeth on individual cusps and testing for biting pain can help identify a cracked tooth or cusp.

thin, narrow and able to be accurately placed. Should difficulties be experienced in identifying a tooth that is sensitive to biting pressure, identification of the tooth can usually be made if a moistened, folded gauze square (or small triangle of hard card) is placed between the teeth. Then the patient is instructed to clench firmly, hold for several seconds and then quickly release. Using this method, the tooth that is sensitive to biting can be readily determined (or at least narrowed down to two opposing teeth). Having the patient clench their teeth and move their lower jaw slightly from side to side while the teeth are still clenched together can also be useful in eliciting a response and identifying the cracked tooth or cusp.

NOTES: Cracked teeth respond better to bite testing *when the teeth are wet*, because the pain produced is due to fluid movement in the dentinal tubules.

Pain on release of pressure is diagnostic of a cracked tooth or a loose restoration, such as a debonded composite resin restoration.

Tooth mobility

Mobility is usually not a good predictor of dental pain. By the time the tooth becomes mobile, there are usually other signs and symptoms that assist in making the diagnosis. Tooth mobility can be a sign of *occlusal trauma*. To check for occlusal trauma, ask the patient to clench together, then place a finger on the suspect tooth and ask the patient to grind slightly. If the tooth moves slightly, but the adjacent teeth do not, the tooth is likely in traumatic occlusion. From a diagnostic perspective, assessment of mobility can be important as there are serious conditions that need to be considered if a tooth *suddenly becomes mobile for no apparent reason.*

Selective anaesthesia

Selectively anesthetizing a tooth, several teeth or an arch may be helpful in identifying a painful tooth, as a means of excluding certain teeth as the source of pain, or as a means of confirming that pain is arising from a particular site. Selective anesthesia is especially useful if there is confusion regarding the arch in which the sensitive tooth is located.

It will only be effective if the anesthetic solution is injected into the site that is the source of the pain. This may not be the site where the pain is experienced. When anaesthetizing an aching tooth (source of the pain), relief is often experienced first at the source of the pain, and then secondly at the site to which the pain is referred. A thorough understanding of the innervation of teeth, especially in the maxillary arch, is essential in accurately interpreting these test results.

If the administration of local anesthetic provides pain relief for only a short period of time (minutes in a patient who presents with chronic pain), it is likely that the patient is suffering from pain of non-dental origin or pain which has a strong psychological basis, for example trigeminal neuropathic orofacial pain (see Chapter 22). Selective anesthesia can also be useful in determining whether pain is caused by a sinusitis.

Muscle pain and selective anaesthesia

Selective anesthesia is useful in the differentiation between dental pain and muscle dysfunction as dental block and infiltration anesthesia will alleviate dental pain but not muscle pain. Those with muscle pain (myofascial pain) often present with a firm taut band of muscle, which is tender on palpation. Injection of 4–5 ml of 2% lignocaine or 3% mepivacaine local anesthetic solution (without adrenaline) into such a trigger point produces immediate relief and is diagnostic of muscle pain.[81]

The application of topical anesthetic will temporarily relieve superficial soft tissue pain, including superficial neuropathic facial pain in some circumstances. Gargling with solutions containing topical anesthetics can temporarily relieve pain on swallowing from glossopharyngeal neuralgia, which presents as severe pain in tonsil and ear. The pain in glossopharyngeal neuralgia is usually triggered by yawning or swallowing and can be confused as arising from the TMJ or masticatory muscles.[82]

Transillumination

Transillumination of teeth with a fiber-optic light (Fig. 11-12) is useful in the initial search for a painful tooth. Discolored teeth have an altered translucency or are virtually opaque, and they can be easily identified by transillumination and then investigated further as a causative factor for a patient's pain. Transillumination is also very helpful in determining the presence of a crack. A crack that extends through the enamel and into the dentin will stop the passage of light from one side of the crack to the other. A crack confined only to the enamel (infraction or craze line) will still permit light to be transmitted from the tooth

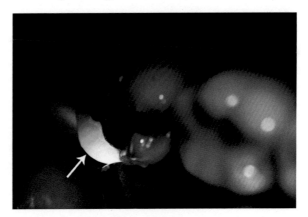

Fig. 11-12 Transillumination with a bright light is a useful mechanism for viewing cracked or discolored tooth structure. A cracked cusp (arrow) can be easily identified using transillumination.

(A)

(B)

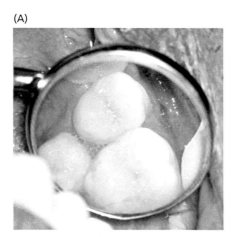

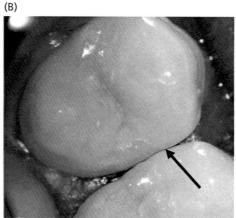

Fig. 11-13 Visualization of a tooth without magnification (A) may not show the cracked tooth structure that is evident on the distal marginal ridge under an operating microscope (arrow) (B).

structure on one side of the crack where the transilluminating light is placed to the tooth structure on the other side of the crack.

Persistent dentin hypersensitivity, which does not respond to conservative measures including desensitizing agents, should raise the clinician's suspicion that a crack may be the cause of the patient's complaint. Further investigation is warranted using magnification and transillumination. Due to the reflection of the light from the cracked surface, a cracked cusp will "light up" with a bright light. The cracks will appear as distinct dark lines in an otherwise bright structure on one side of the crack. Cracked teeth can present with bizarre symptoms and a prolonged history of pain.

Magnification

The role of magnification in detecting an offending tooth is often underestimated (Fig. 11-13). Magnifying loupes or a surgical operating microscope help to reveal open restoration margins, subtle non-carious cervical lesions or cracked cusps which may not be apparent with the naked eye.

Test cavity

A test cavity involves drilling a small cavity in the occlusal aspect of the tooth up until the dentin is reached without use of local anesthesia. If the innervation of the pulp is intact, the patient will complain of pain. The prepared cavity is then restored as the pulp is deemed vital. In case of lack of response, the preparation is deepened and an absolute lack of response is typical of necrotic pulp.

Drilling a test cavity is particularly useful when there is a full crown restoration and all the pulp tests inconclusive. The prepared cavity can also be used to place the tip of an electric pulp tester if access to sound tooth structure is limited due to the presence of crown.[83] A test cavity can be prepared: a) to evaluate if there is a response to drilling and/or b) to make room for a pulp-testing device to make contact with dentin. It is important to remember that although this testing is particularly useful in identifying the cause of pain, it is limited to situations where the pulpal status of a tooth is in question.

Ultrasound

The utility of ultrasound in diagnosis of orofacial pain is limited to detecting changes in the temporomandibular joint, measuring the thickness of masticatory muscles (especially the masseter) and detecting other non-dental, soft tissue head and neck pathology (cysts and salivary gland disturbances).[84] Ultrasound has little use in routine orofacial pain diagnosis.

Chapter 12

Diagnosing Dental Pain

Alex J. Moule and Unni Krishnan

Introduction

Orofacial pain can result from a large number of causes. However, by far the greatest amount of acute orofacial pain has a dental origin.[85] Although signs and symptoms can vary considerably from person to person and from tooth to tooth, without intervention, pain of dental origin generally proceeds along a fairly predictable path from initiation of symptoms, to pulp necrosis and to the development of symptoms of periapical infection.

To appreciate mechanisms of pain arising from the dental pulps, an understanding of its origins is required.[86] In summary, two types of pain arise from the pulp, mediated by different nerve fibers, each with their own individual characteristics. The first is mediated by A delta fibers, which transmit short, sharp fast pain, often induced by stimuli such as cold, heat, air, mechanical stimulation (drilling) and osmotic stimuli. Pain is initiated in the pulp by a rapid fluid flow in dentinal tubules. Once the affected tooth and the exposed dentin are identified, this type of pain can usually be treated by sealing the exposed tubules.

A second type of pain is mediated by C-type fibers and is usually experienced as a slow, dull, aching and poorly localized pain. Pain fibers are activated by stimuli that are noxious to the pulp, including inflammatory mediators (pulpitis). Severe pain of this character can be difficult to diagnose and generally indicates serious inflammatory damage (irreversible pulpitis) necessitating endodontic therapy or removal of the tooth.[86] A characteristic of pulpitis is that the pain is not constant, but changes over time. It can also be referred to a more remote site in the jaw, or to a site in the opposing arch but only on the same side as the offending tooth. It is not referred across the midline.

While previous studies have failed to show any major clinical correlation between presenting signs and symptoms and the histological state of the pulp,[87] more recent investigations using contemporary techniques claim to show a significant correlation between current clinical diagnostic criteria and histology.[88]

From a treatment perspective, pulpal pain is broadly classified as suffering reversible inflammation, which can be alleviated by treatment (*reversible pulpitis*); irreversible inflammation, which cannot be treated conservatively (*irreversible pulpitis*); and pulp necrosis, where death of all or part of the pulp has occurred. While guidelines exist to help differentiate between these, and pain profiles are attributed to each stage, most clinicians would agree that the boundaries between these are often blurred.[89] Notwithstanding the above, and acknowledging that 40% of a pulp may become necrotic without first becoming symptomatic,[90] symptomatically *the progression of dental pain from initial symptoms to pulp necrosis and infection is a continuum with a variable time frame.*

Clinical progression of pulpal disease

From a clinical perspective, pain from the dental pulp develops progressively through this continuum in which various phases can be identified, although the boundaries between them cannot be. Not all teeth pass noticeably through each phase, and not all teeth behave in the same manner; therefore, individual variations are immense. What is reasonably constant, however, is the forward progression from one symptomatic phase to another. An understanding of these phases is needed in any discussion on pain diagnosis, particularly when considering whether a particular pain source is or is not of dental origin. Treatment categories are a separate and simpler issue and are not discussed in this manual.

Diagnosing Dental and Orofacial Pain: A Clinical Manual, First Edition. Edited by Alex J. Moule and M. Lamar Hicks.
© 2017 John Wiley & Sons, Ltd. Published 2017 by John Wiley & Sons, Ltd.
Companion website: www.wiley.com/go/moule/dental_and_orofacial_pain

Phase 1

The tooth becomes sensitive to thermal stimulations and possibly to sweetness. The pain is of short, sharp momentary duration and occurs only when stimulated ("*ouch and gone*"). This stage may last for weeks or even years. Pulp sensibility testing will be positive. There may be a transient exaggerated response to cold, but no radiographic evidence of changes.

Phase 2

The severity of response to thermal stimuli increases. There may be an exaggerated response to cold. Response to stimuli may be quite severe, but still dissipates quickly. There may be a lingering awareness, but just for a few more seconds after the stimulus. There is no radiographic evidence of periradicular changes. Tooth identification is best achieved by the use of cold or hot water under rubber dam.

A factor that is often ignored, in determining whether pulpitis is reversible or irreversible, is *whether or not the cause of the pain can be eliminated.* With treatment, it is possible that pulpal inflammation can be reversed (reversible pulpitis). If the cause is not eliminated, progression will be towards irreversible pulpitis and its consequences. If the cause can be isolated and treated, there is a greater chance that pulpal inflammation will resolve (reverse).

Thus, pain associated with a deep carious lesion is more likely to resolve, and the pulp more likely to return to a healthy state if the lesion is treated, than pain in a heavily restored tooth in which the cause of the pain cannot be detected.[91] There is recent histological evidence that initial pulpal reaction to caries is initially limited to the focal accumulation of inflammatory cells near the affected odontoblasts and the pulpal parenchyma is unaffected.[92] However, there is still limited evidence for clinical correlation.

NOTE: A non-carious heavily restored tooth that becomes *symptomatic* without an obvious reason is likely cracked. Whenever reviewing pain in restored teeth, consider:

What has changed to make this tooth now become symptomatic?

Phase 3

Response to stimuli becomes more severe and the ensuing pain is not resolved quickly over time. The pulp is likely irreversibly damaged (irreversible pulpitis). The severe pain may last minutes or even hours after stimulation. There is a lingering and exaggerated response to both cold and heat, but no radiographic evidence of periradicular changes. Teeth may remain symptomatic for hours or weeks. As the tooth is still responsive to thermal stimulus (and unless the patient still reports severe sensitivity to cold), tooth identification is best achieved by the use of hot water under rubber dam isolation.

Phase 4

A recurrent constant, severe, unrelenting toothache develops. This may be prolonged after stimulation or may be spontaneous. From a pain diagnosis point of view, it is important to understand that (in contrast to other types of pain conditions) *with acute pulpal pain (toothache), the intensity and character change over time.* That is, the pain levels do not remain constant at the same intensity for long periods of time. Rather, pain ebbs and flows (waves of pain), at times becoming very severe, particularly on stimulation; other times less so. The pain may wake the patient at night and prevent them from sleeping. Some patients may experience extreme sensitivity to thermal changes that may last for hours. Analgesia is difficult to obtain. Some tenderness to percussion may be present. The pulp will not usually respond to conservative treatment.

If untreated, severe pain (with some exceptions, e.g. cracked teeth with large pulps) will usually only last for a number of days. Then pulpal necrosis occurs, and thereafter the pain can stop abruptly. Tooth identification is sometimes difficult, as responses to thermal stimuli may be equivocal. Pain may be referred to a distant site or to a different arch. *Thus the site of pain may no longer be the source of the pain.*

There may be a lingering and exaggerated response to heat, but only at the source of the pain. A slight widening of the periodontal ligament may be apparent, but the lamina dura is usually intact. Where pain is referred, the teeth at the site of pain will respond normally to pulp sensibility testing.

Not all teeth at this phase respond to cold stimulation, but *all teeth with pulpitis respond to the heat.* Indeed, some are relieved by the application of cold. Thus tooth identification can be best achieved with using hot water under rubber dam isolation.

Phase 5

Pain may cease completely. This is due to the fact that all (or part) of the pulp becomes necrotic. The pulp may no longer respond immediately to thermal stimuli. However, a *prolonged and delayed response to the application of heat* may be present. On such stimulation, the pain may last for hours. Pain on percussion may or may not be present. *Demonstrable radiographic changes may, however, not be evident for days after pulp necrosis has occurred.* Later on, radiographic changes (widening of the periodontal ligament space, or apical loss of the lamina dura) become evident.

Thus, while radiographic changes may not be seen clearly at the time of the initial complaint of pain, changes may be demonstrable on a film taken a short time later. A new radiographic examination is therefore justified a short time after an initial consultation if pain persists.

NOTE: Before viewing any radiograph, check the date it was taken.

Phase 6

Periapical pain responses develop as part of, or overlapping, the above. Once necrosis develops, the host responses and immune system play a role in the progression of symptoms. Necrotic teeth can remain symptom free for a variable length of time. In the usual turn of events after irreversible pulpitis, the tooth shortly becomes sensitive to biting forces and to percussion (although, anecdotally, biting on a tooth in the early stages of this phase can produce some pain relief). Sensitivity to pressure may become acute. Ultimately, biting pressure may cause severe and prolonged pain.

The tooth is non-responsive to pulp sensibility testing. Thus pulp sensibility testing is a useful means of excluding adjacent teeth as the cause. Tooth identification is made easier by a positive response to percussion, lack of response to pulp sensibility testing, and concomitant radiographic changes.

NOTE: Of note is that pulp necrosis can occur without being painful at first and that necrosis is not synonymous with symptoms. Thus the *presence of a periapical radiolucency is not an indication that a particular tooth is the cause of a patient's discomfort.* Mistakes are commonly made when practitioners try to diagnose only from a radiograph. Radiography is an adjunct to diagnosis. The history has to match the radiographic findings.

Phase 7

Symptoms of severe periapical inflammation develop. The severity of the local responses is dependent on host responses and also virulence of the bacteria. The tooth can become extruded, mobile and painful to touch, and surrounding tissues may become swollen. The amount of pain experienced is ultimately dependent on whether drainage occurs. Where drainage occurs spontaneously (via a fistulous tract), symptoms can quickly resolve or diminish. A chronic abscess develops. Pain relief can be obtained by surgical drainage or by antibiotic therapy. In these cases relief may be temporary and pain will likely return over time.

Where drainage occurs into soft tissue, swelling may predominate, but pain can be less intense. Where there is no drainage, particularly in the case of infected maxillary lateral incisors and lower premolar and molar teeth where the thickness of the buccal plate can confine the infection, pain will predominate and can be intense. Where drainage occurs sublingually the airway may be compromised, a life-threatening emergency.

Long-standing infections, and/or dental infections in patients with medical problems or who are immunocompromised, can lead to osteomyelitis. Tooth identification is generally easy as the tooth is locally sensitive. Radiographic changes are evident, which include loss of the lamina dura and periapical radiolucency in the surrounding apical bone. The tooth will not respond to thermal testing. Pulp sensibility testing is a useful tool to exclude adjacent non-involved teeth.

Phase 8

Systemic symptoms may develop. The patient may become unwell and febrile. Antibiotic therapy is warranted. Antibiotics are essential in the treatment of a periapical abscess that does not drain; for patients who develop systemic symptoms; for patients who have facial swelling, particularly in the anterior maxilla; and for patients who are immunocompromised or who have medical conditions that affect their ability to respond to infections.

NOTE: There is no indication to prescribe antibiotics for a painful vital tooth or teeth which are temperature sensitive.

Left untreated, the patient will continue to experience pain and swelling, and develop systemic symptoms, which at times can be life threatening, particularly in mandibular molars where sublingual swelling compromises the airway, and where infections in the anterior mid-face pass directly into the brain because of the venous communication between the facial vein and cavernous sinus through the ophthalmic vein.

Confirmatory tests for dental pain

Most orofacial pain is of dental origin. Thus an assumption can first be made that orofacial pain is *dental*, until history, descriptors and tests prove otherwise. Nevertheless, diagnostic errors are regularly made if the possibility of a non-dental cause is not countenanced. The patterns of dental pain are reasonably clear, as are the many patterns of pain that are non-dental.

It is the philosophy of this manual that *history taking is more important than testing*, and that if clinicians take an accurate history, listen to the descriptors, and use screening questions to pass up and across a diagnostic tree, errors in diagnosis should not occur. Indeed, it is estimated that over 80% of clinical diagnosis are based on history alone. Clinical examination contributes to a further 5 to 10%, and the remainder are investigations and special tests.[93] Once a probable diagnosis of dental pain is formulated, there are many individual tests for examining the status of the pulps in teeth and to confirm a diagnosis (see Chapter 12).

NOTE: Objective testing is carried out to confirm a probable diagnosis or exclude possibilities in a differential or probable diagnosis.

An inadequate demonstrable local dental cause for the pain should be a red flag in the diagnostic process, as is the patient's use of descriptors that do not add up for dental pain. In the absence of signs and symptoms that confirm dental pathology, in particular the stimulated nature of the pain, the clinical and radiographic evidence of infection and confirmatory responses to testing, a dental cause is not confirmed. A diagnosis of dental involvement should only be made if there is at least a positive history and two independent signs and symptoms that confirm each case.

Treatment considerations

It is beyond the scope of this manual to discuss treatment options for teeth causing dental pain. There are numerous endodontic texts that describe treatment in detail.[94,95] In principle, however, treatment is directed first to control of pain and control of infection. No treatment should be carried out without a confirmed pulpal and periapical diagnosis. No treatment should be undertaken if clinical diagnosis testing is inconclusive and does not match the diagnosis. There are many classifications that have been used for pulpal and periapical diagnosis designed to assist clinicians making treatment decisions.[89]

Some useful questions if a dental cause is suspected

NOTE: Not all these questions are necessary when diagnosing most dental pain. Usually, dental pain follows a predictable path and is easy to diagnose and treat. In difficult-to-diagnose cases, however, more detailed questioning is required:

1. *What sort of pain are you having?*
   Consider whether the pain follows a dental pain pattern and whether the descriptors are appropriate (see Chapter 5); for example, constant, burning, non-pulsatile toothaches are non-dental in origin. Constant non-variable toothaches are also unlikely to be of dental origin.
2. *Do you have any sensitivity to cold, heat or sweetness?*
   Almost invariably, temperature sensitivity indicates the pain is of dental origin. Exceptions to this are maxillary teeth in a patient with maxillary sinusitis, and teeth of patients in the early stages of pre-trigeminal neuralgia (teeth can be temperature sensitive, but the descriptors used by the patient are usually different). *Pain to sweetness is invariably tooth pain.*
3. *Is there anything that makes the pain worse or better?*
   Look here for thermal stimulus, pain on biting, pain on change of posture, lying down, sitting up response to medications and so on (see Chapter 11).

NOTE: Almost all dental pain can be controlled by normal analgesia. Take note if regular analgesics do not change the character of the pain, and if other medication, such as muscle relaxants, is more effective.

4. *(If stimulated) Is this "ouch and gone" pain or "ouch and stay" pain?*
   How this question is phrased will depend on individual practitioners. What is important is to determine how long the pain remains after stimulation. *Ouch and gone* pain is usually a sign of reversible pulpitis. Depending on the length of time the pain lasts after the stimulus, *ouch and stay* pain is usually a sign of irreversible pulpitis. For tooth pain, the longer the pain lasts after stimulation (*ouch and stay*), the more likely the condition is irreversible.
5. *How has the pain changed over time?*
   Dental pain follows a pattern that usually develops in a progression of stages. A characteristic of pulpitis is that the pain is not constant but changes over time. Constant non-pulsatile pain is not characteristic of pulpal pain.
6. *Have you had pain on the other side of the mouth?*
   Bilateral pain is not dental pain. Bilateral pain is not referred pain from teeth.
7. *Have you had this sort of pain before, and have you been treated for this?*
   This question should assist the patient to recount past similar pain experiences that may not have been remembered in the initial description of the pain. Patients with pulpitis can report that they had thermal sensitivity in the past. Patients may give a history of past treatment which may or may not have been successful. Spontaneous *multiple* toothaches are unlikely to be of dental origin.
8. *Has the treatment you have received changed the character of the pain you have been experiencing?*
   If the patient has dental pain, the treatment carried out should change the character of the pain. If not, the wrong tooth may have been treated or the pain is of non-dental origin.
9. *Does anything make your teeth hurt, or does the tooth start hurting by itself?*
   Spontaneous dental pain is more likely to be a sign of irreversible pulpitis.
10. *Where is the pain? Can you put your finger on where the pain is?*
    Is the manner in which the patient explains the site of the pain consistent with dental pain (see Chapter 4)?
11. *Where did the pain start?*
    Pain may be referred from one tooth to another site, the site of referral being different from the source of pain. However, the site where the pain is first noted is more likely to reflect the source of the pain.
12. *When did the pain start?*
    Can the patient tell you with any certainty when the pain problems commenced and whether there were any circumstances (e.g. recent restorative

procedures) associated with its commencement, including dental treatment and trauma?

13. *How long have you been in pain?*
Dental pain usually follows a distinct pattern. With the possible exception of cracked teeth, acute pulpitis usually lasts for no more than a few days to a week, not years. Consider a non-dental cause if the pain has been present for months or years.

14. *Are any of your teeth sore to bite on?*
Sensitivity to biting can be due to a number of dental causes. Dental infection is only one of these. Pulp sensibility testing must be carried out for any tooth that is sensitive to biting pressure. The quality of the pain can assist with the diagnosis (e.g. very sharp pain may indicate a cracked tooth). However, take care with your diagnosis if more than one tooth is sensitive to biting or percussion, as a non-dental cause has to be considered.

15. *Have you been able to sleep?*
Patients with tooth pain that has prevented them from sleeping are likely have an irreversible pulpitis or necrotic pulp.

16. *Does it hurt to press over the top of any teeth?*
This assists in the identification of a symptomatic non-vital tooth and/or to identify periapical infection.

17. *Have you had any soft tissue swelling or tenderness in the area?*
A past history of soft tissue swelling helps to confirm a dental cause if reported in the presence of signs and symptoms of dental disease. The location of the swelling is important to note. Dental pathosis is not the only cause of orofacial soft tissue swelling. Lymph node and salivary gland pathology, and trigeminal neuropathic pain, can present with significant orofacial swelling.

18. *Does it hurt to press on the side of your face?*
In the absence of demonstrable intraoral dental pathology, pain to pressing on the side of the face is an indication of a non-dental problem, often muscle pain.

Referral of dental pain

As mentioned previously, dental pain can also be referred to another tooth or to a more remote site in the jaw or to an opposing arch, but only on the same side as the offending tooth. When referral occurs, diagnosis can be more difficult. The site to which the pain is referred appears devoid of any signs of inflammation infection. Objective testing, such as pulp sensibility testing of the tooth, will show normal pulpal status.

Referred pain or *heterotrophic pain* is that pain which is felt at a place distant from the one causing the pain.[96] This can be confusing for the clinician and the patient, as the site to which the pain has been referred is not the source of the discomfort, and will be normal and devoid of any disease. Referral of pain

occurs as a result of one or a combination of factors. Understanding the patterns of referral helps to explain the confusing nature of heterotrophic pain.

Pain is usually referred in a cephalic direction (towards the cranium)

This means pain originating from the sacral region, often referred to lumbar, lumbar to thoracic, thoracic to cervical and cervical to trigeminal.[96] In other words, it is more common for pain originating from, say, neck muscles to radiate to the orofacial region rather than the other way around.[96] Thus it is common for mandibular molar pulpitis pain to be referred to maxillary molar teeth following this cephalic pattern. Such pain is not relieved by anesthetic blocking of the tooth or the site where the pain is felt, but anesthetizing the trigger point will relieve the pain. Pain referral patterns for muscles to the orofacial region are described in Chapters 14 and 15.

Convergence of neurons occurs from same region in the trigeminal spinal nucleus

One of the reasons why identification of the origin of dental pain is difficult is because of the convergence of neurons from multiple teeth pulp onto the same region in the trigeminal spinal nucleus.[97] This results in multiple afferent neurons from pulp synapsing with a single projection that form the trigeminothalamic tract, causing pain to radiate to areas beyond the region of injury (Fig. 12-1). Thus, pain from acute pulpitis can often be poorly localized and diffuse. In addition, the dental pulp lacks proprioceptive fibers which provide the sense of location, also making it difficult for the patient to locate the offending tooth.[98]

Vertical lamination pattern of representation in the spinal trigeminal

There is a vertical lamination pattern of representation as well in the spinal trigeminal nucleus, with structures close to the midline (anterior teeth) being represented at a cephalic position and those from the lateral aspect (posterior teeth) terminating at the caudal part of the nucleus (Fig. 12-2).[96] It is therefore common to see pain from a molar being referred to canine and canine to incisors in the same arch.[96]

Peripheral and central sensitization

Processing of afferent impulses is not static. Responses to afferent input are altered after persistent activation. This is manifested by an increased sensitivity of the neurons and an expansion of their responsive fields.[99] From a clinical perspective, the longer a painful situation (toothache) is present, the greater the reduction in the sensitivity threshold and the more responsive the sensory neuron will become to

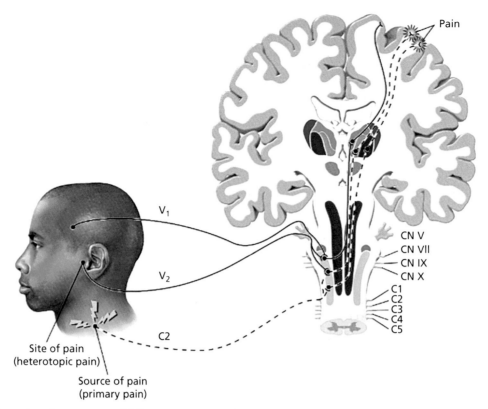

Fig. 12-1 Illustration of convergence of different neurons onto the same second-order neurons of the trigeminothalamic tract (adapted from *Cohen's Pathways of Pulp Tenth*, ed. St Loius Missouri: Mosby Elsevier; 2011 with permission).

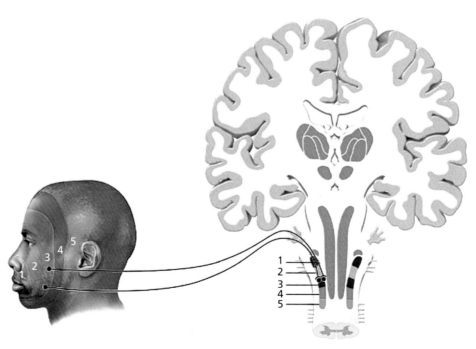

Fig. 12-2 The laminated pattern of representation of orofacial structures in the trigeminal spinal nucleus. Note the cephalic position of the structures close to midline and caudal position of lateral structures (adapted from *Cohen's Pathways of Pulp Tenth*, ed. St Loius Missouri: Mosby Elsevier; 2011 with permission).

stimulation, also with a wider field of sensitivity. As a consequence, pain referral will occur more frequently and more widely, the longer a painful stimulus is present. Central sensitization, which can result in the development of neuropathic pain, occurs in the same manner (see Chapter 22).

Most frequently referred pain occurs within a single nerve root

Most frequently referred pain occurs within a single nerve root. The trigeminal nerve has three main branches. Pain originating from one branch could be passed on to another; for example, pain from a mandibular molar can be referred from the *mandibular* branch of the trigeminal nerve to the maxillary branch of the trigeminal nerve, but within the same nerve root, and the patient could perceive pain in the areas innervated by the *maxillary* branch of the same nerve.[96] It is also common for pain from mandibular molars (inferior alveolar branch) to be referred to the auricular branch of the same division of the nerve. Referred dental pain never crosses the midline in the orofacial region (unless it is originating in the midline). The exception is cervical spinal pain, which can at times be referred across the midline.[96]

In summary, though referred pain usually follows a cephalic direction, a posterior-to-anterior pattern of referral should also be considered when confronted with dental pain. The following questions should help in asserting whether a referred pain is involved or not.

Confirmatory tests and findings

An important differentiating factor in diagnosing referred pain is that provoking the region where the pain is felt does not increase or reproduce the pain. Conversely, stimulation of the source of the pain will stimulate pain in the site of referral. In addition, local anesthetic placed at the **site** of the pain will not alleviate the pain. This only occurs if the local anesthetic is placed at the *source* of the pain, for example the aching tooth or trigger point of the muscle.

Questions to ask if referred pain is suspected

Where did you first feel the pain?

Patients can usually locate the pain accurately when they first feel the sensation. It is when the intensity increases that they are unable to determine the location. The position where the pain is first felt more commonly reflects the source of the pain.

Is the pain superficial or deep?

Superficial pain is unlikely to be involved in referred pain. So if the patient is insisting that the pain is *superficial and spreading*, it is more likely to be from a neurogenic source (herpes zoster, postherpetic neuralgia, peripheral neuritis, paroxysmal neuralgia etc.) rather than of cutaneous origin. If the pain is deep and localizable when provoked, it is likely to be of musculoskeletal origin.

Can you localize the pain? Is the pain localized or diffuse?

Pain that is deep and diffuse usually arises from deep somatic tissue such as cardiac or dental pulp, though occasionally musculoskeletal pain can be deep and diffuse. This is because the pain-producing nociceptors from both skeletal muscle and visceral structure do converge in the central nervous system.

Where did the pain first start?

Pain referral is usually a secondary process. Thus the place where the pain first started is more likely to be the source of the pain.

Chapter 13

Diagnosing Cracked (Crown Fractured) Teeth

Alex J. Moule

Cracked (crown fractured) teeth

It is well known that cracked or incompletely fractured teeth can become symptomatic, often resulting in a protracted history of pain of varying intensity. These teeth may present a wide range of symptoms, from occasional discomfort to severe and prolonged pain, especially if the pulp in the tooth is large.[100] Intermittent pain on biting and sensitivity to cold are the most consistent complaints.[101] However, teeth with cracks can produce some of the most bizarre symptoms encountered in practice. The source of the pain may be difficult to locate.

Classically, the symptoms are:

- Pain on biting, particularly when biting on hard food or a small seed
- Sensitivity to thermal changes, especially cold.[101,102]

RULE OF THUMB: An unexplained *dental* pain equals a cracked tooth until proven otherwise.

NOTES:
- *Long-term unexplained orofacial pain, including severe pulpitis, can be caused by cracks in teeth.* Thus it is important to examine all teeth carefully under magnification and illumination when diagnosing patients with chronic orofacial pain, to eliminate fractured teeth as a source of the complaint.
- If a composite resin restoration debonds, symptoms may mimic those of a cracked tooth. In these cases pressure applied to the restoration produces sensitivity, but not when applied to the surrounding tooth structure.
- Pain from a cracked cusp invariably resolves if the cusp separates (fractures) from the tooth.

Risk sites

Teeth can crack through the crown; however, cracks often only involve cusps. *Cuspal fractures* are most commonly found in mandibular molars, followed in descending order by maxillary premolars, maxillary molars and then mandibular premolars. In mandibular molars, the lingual cusps are the most commonly involved. In maxillary molars and premolars, cracked buccal cusps predominate (Fig. 13-1). Non-functional cusps are more commonly cracked than functional cusps.[103,104]

Of note in diagnosis, if a cracked tooth hurts every time the patient bites, the problem cusp is usually a working cusp. If it only hurts occasionally, it is likely a non-working cusp.

Questions to ask: *When does the tooth hurt? Does it hurt every time you bite or only sometimes?*

Cause of pain

Although it has been postulated that "crack propagation" is the initiating cause of pain in fractured teeth, there are no data to support this proposition. There are no evidence-based data on the manner in which cracks occur in crowns of teeth and how they propagate. It is likely, though, that in cuspal cracks the dentin fractures from the pulpo-axial line angle to the dentino-enamel junction in a single incident.[105] Pain on stimulation is most likely due to fluid movement in dentinal tubules as the crack is activated.[106] Ingress of bacteria (microleakage) through the crack, and into the dentinal tubules and then the pulp, has been implicated in the development of pulpitis in fractured teeth.[105]

Diagnosing Dental and Orofacial Pain: A Clinical Manual, First Edition. Edited by Alex J. Moule and M. Lamar Hicks.
© 2017 John Wiley & Sons, Ltd. Published 2017 by John Wiley & Sons, Ltd.
Companion website: www.wiley.com/go/moule/dental_and_orofacial_pain

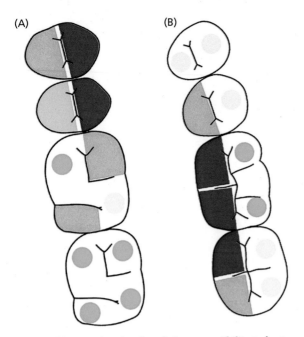

(A) (B)

Fig. 13-1 Diagram showing the relative susceptibility to fracture of the cusps in maxillary and mandibular premolar and molar teeth. Red cusps are the most susceptible, followed by orange and blue. Green dots indicate low risk areas, and yellow very low (courtesy of Dr Graham Craig, Dental Outlook, Australia).

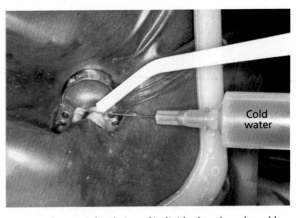

Fig. 13-2 Sequential isolation of individual teeth under rubber dam and testing with cold water will rapidly identify a cold-sensitive cracked tooth. Allow the water to pool over the whole tooth surface.

Management of cracked teeth

The diagnosis and management of a cracked tooth are simplified if a four-stage process is followed:

1. Tooth identification
2. Crack confirmation
3. Crack investigation
4. Treatment planning.

1. Tooth identification

Tooth identification is often easy. The patient is aware of the offending tooth, a crack can be seen, and the cracked cusp is easily identified. In some teeth, however, tooth identification is more difficult and requires additional investigation.

In considering cracked teeth, there is a BIG difference between *pulp sensibility testing* and *tooth identification*. Pulp sensibility testing is used to determine whether a pulp is responsive to a thermal or electric stimulus. Testing every tooth in the arch with a cold stimulus or an electric pulp tester is often inconclusive, as the crack may not be activated during these tests. *Tooth identification,* in contrast, requires only the identification of the painful tooth and involves reproducing the patient's chief complaint by applying the stimulus that causes the complaint (e.g. sweets, cold fluids, hot foods or biting). For a tooth with a crack, this means testing with cold fluids and/or with biting pressure.

Testing each tooth on the affected side with ice-cold water *under rubber dam isolation* is an effective way of establishing which tooth is the temperature-sensitive

cracked tooth (Fig. 13-2) (see Chapter 11). This testing is more accurate than refrigerant sprays, as it allows the cold fluid to pool over the crack and to initiate the pain response.

2. Crack confirmation

Once the identity of the symptomatic tooth has been established, it is necessary to confirm that a crack is present. Cracks can be identified by direct vision, by bite testing or by using selective percussion, controlled wedging, clamping, staining or occasionally radiographic examination.

Direct vision

Direct vision with a bright (fiber-optic) light may show the following:

Cracks in the enamel

It is not uncommon for teeth to show vertical enamel fracture lines (craze lines or infractions), particularly in teeth under load. These are usually not clinically important. However, any crack line that runs in a direction other than vertical is an important indicator that a crack is present (Fig. 13-3) and that it involves the entire cusp.

A vertical crack in enamel that is "notched" on the incisal edge or occlusal cusp tip is also an important indicator of underlying cracked tooth structure (Fig. 13-4).

Cracks on the marginal ridges

A line running across a marginal ridge is a sign that the tooth has a crack. The crack may or may not be stained. A crack involving a marginal ridge can appear (in order of severity) as a single dark line, as a double black line or as a double black line separated by a yellowish brown line. Occasionally, the crack appears as a white frosted line between two

(A)   (B)

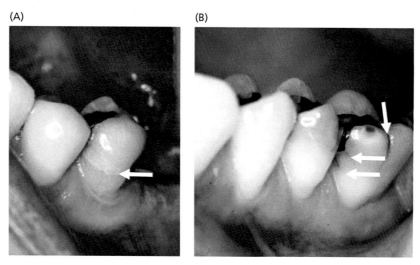

Fig. 13-3 A mandibular premolar tooth (A) exhibiting a crack running horizontally from the floor of the box from across the buccal cusp (arrowed). A mandibular first molar (B) with cracks emanating from corners of a cavity preparation (horizontal arrows) and a crack in the buccal groove, signs that the buccal cusp is completely cracked.

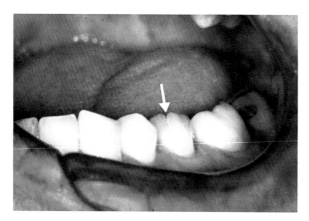

Fig. 13-4 A mandibular premolar with a notched vertical crack (arrow) indicating that the tooth is severely fractured.

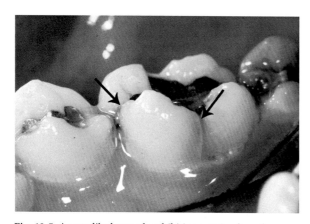

Fig. 13-5 A mandibular tooth exhibiting a stained crack running across the mesial marginal ridge and a vertical crack running between the two lingual cusps (arrows).

stained lines. A clear crack may indicate that only a cusp is cracked.

Unless the tooth is cracked mesiodistally, a crack on a marginal ridge is almost always accompanied by a second crack bucco-lingually between two cusps (Fig. 13-5). If there is a crack on a marginal ridge in a restored tooth *and* a crack between the two lingual cusps, one cusp is cracked. If both marginal ridges are cracked, both cusps are cracked, or the crack passes through the body of the tooth.

Cracks in the access closure filling

If a mesiodistal crack is seen in a temporary filling placed in the access opening of a tooth being endodontically treated, the tooth is undoubtedly cracked. While it is common for unsupported temporary filling material to crack mesiodistally across a box form, for a crack to occur bucco-lingually in a temporary filling that is surrounded by tooth structure, the underlying tooth structure also has to be cracked (Fig. 13-6). Of note, it has been shown that some hygroscopic temporary restorative materials can expand on setting by up to 20%. *In vitro* this has been associated with fractures of tooth structure when this material is used as a temporary restoration in endodontic access preparations.[107]

Color changes in cusps

In direct bright light a cracked cusp may appear brighter and more radio-opaque than its uncracked counterparts. In the shadow, it will appear darker (Figs 13-7 A, B and C).

Changes in the marginal definition

Changes in the marginal definition between tooth structure and an adjacent restoration may be an indication that the tooth is cracked. This may appear as a frosted edge on the enamel margin adjacent to the restoration (Fig. 13-8).

Transillumination

Holding a bright (fiber-optic) light at alternately different angles against a tooth is an excellent means of demonstrating cracks in teeth. A cracked

(A)   (B)

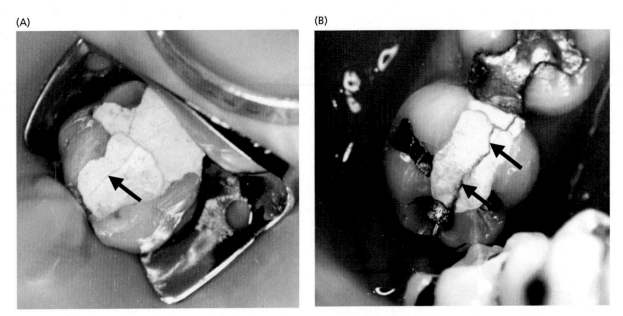

Fig. 13-6 When a mesiodistal crack is seen in a endodontic access closure, it is confirmation that the tooth structure is cracked. In (A), the access closure is cracked in a number of places. While unsupported temporary filling material can crack, the mesiodistal crack (arrow) is a sign that the underlying tooth is cracked. In (B), (arrows) an obvious mesiodistal crack across the access closure is a sign that the underlying tooth structure is cracked.

(A)   (B)

(C)

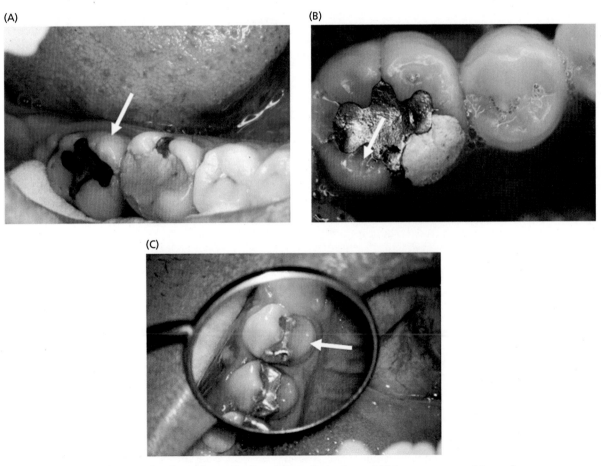

Fig. 13-7 (A) Mandibular second molar with a cracked mesiolingual cusp (arrow). This cusp appears whiter and more opaque than the other cusps. Note the crack across the mesial marginal ridge. (B) Cracked distolingual cusp in a lower molar in shadow appears darker than other cusps. (C) A maxillary first premolar tooth with a cracked palatal cusp. Note the dark color of this cusp compared with the buccal cusp. The adjacent premolar (not arrowed) is root-canal filled and stained.

(A)

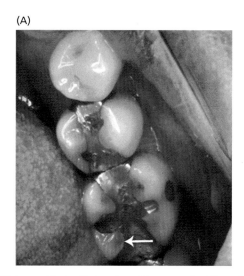

(B)

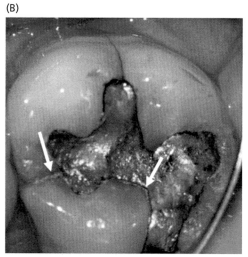

Fig. 13-8 (A) A mandibular first molar with two cracked lingual cusps. Note the loss of marginal definition and a frosty margin between the cusps and the amalgam restoration (arrow). (B) Maxillary molar tooth with a fractured palatal cusp. Note the frosted appearance of the crack line on the mesiopalatal and adjacent to the amalgam restoration.

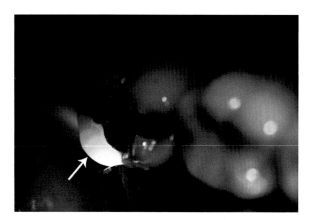

Fig. 13-9 A cracked cusp is clearly visible when a bright (fiber-optic) light is held up against it.

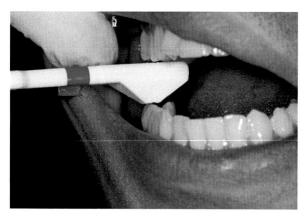

Fig. 13-10 Proprietary products (e.g. Tooth Slooth® or Fractfinder®) are useful for detecting cracks. A folded piece of wet gauze or piece of hard paper card can be useful in diagnostically difficult cases.

cusp is accentuated because the crack stops the light from being transmitted into the adjacent tooth structure. Light is reflected back into the fractured portion, making it appear brighter (Fig. 13-9).

Bite testing

A number of proprietary products, for example Fractfinder® or Tooth Slooth®, are available to help identity cracked teeth (Fig. 13-10). These products are useful in many cases. However, as the maximum intercuspal force occurs when the teeth are together or almost together and decreases markedly as the inter-occlusal distance increases, proprietary products can be too large and hold the teeth too far apart during bite testing, thus preventing sufficient force being applied to predictably activate cracks in the teeth. A piece of wet gauze, folded to a point, or a similarly shaped piece of hard paper card, can be very useful in identifying the presence of a crack. When testing for biting reactions, ensure the teeth are wet.

NOTE: Because pain from a cracked tooth is most likely due to fluid movement in the dentinal tubules, cracked teeth should be tested *wet* and not *dry*.

Selective percussion

Selective percussion (Fig. 13-11), which involves tapping on individual cusps one at a time and assessing the painful response, has been suggested as a method to identify cracked teeth and cusps. This technique is often unreliable because it does not reproduce the environment in which the patient experiences their chief complaint. For selective percussion to be effective, the direction of the percussive blow has to be in a direction that activates the crack. Selective percussion is often ineffective.

Controlled wedging and rebound pain

Controlled wedging, which is the application of sustained pressure on individual cusps followed by rapid release of this pressure, is an effective way to identify a cracked cusp or a cracked tooth (Fig. 13-12). Pain that occurs on release of pressure (*rebound pain*) is a strong indication that the tooth is cracked.[108] The same is true if force is applied to a composite resin restoration that has debonded.

Clamp or retainer test

A response similar to "rebound pain" can be elicited if a rubber dam clamp is placed onto a cracked tooth

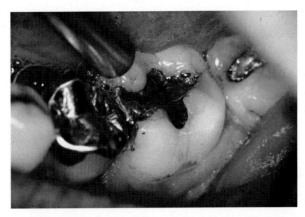

Fig. 13-11 Selective percussion involves tapping on individual cusps with an instrument (e.g. a mirror handle). The direction of the blow must be in a direction that activates the crack.

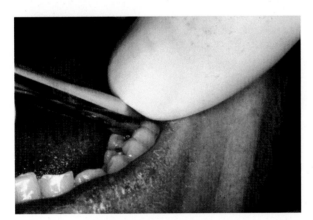

Fig. 13-12 A sustained and controlled wedging force allows individual cusps to be loaded. If rapid release of the force results in *rebound pain*, it is indicative of a crack in the tooth.

for a few seconds and then suddenly removed. Anecdotally this has been termed the *clamp test*. This is a useful test when selective percussion does not elicit a response from a patient who is complaining of cracked tooth pain. It is important to forewarn the patient that they will likely feel a very sharp pain on the release of the clamp. Be sure to ask the patient whether they felt it was a *sharp tooth pain* or discomfort from the clamp impinging on the gum tissue.

Staining

The use of biological stains such as Methylene Blue or vegetable dyes is helpful to visualize a crack (Fig. 13-13).

Radiography

Very few cracks can be seen radiographically. Radiography is only helpful if the direction of the beam is in line or parallel with the direction or plane of the crack or fracture (Fig. 13-14). Because most cracks are mesiodistal or oblique in orientation, they are thus not visible. Radiographs may be suggestive whether a crack is present. When viewing a radiograph of a suspected cracked tooth, the following can be assessed:

- *The presence of dentinal sclerosis*: Teeth with long-standing cracks may show a V-shaped radiopacity in the dentin subjacent to the cracked tooth structure, due to sclerosis of dentinal tubules.
- *The presence of horizontal bone loss*: Isolated horizontal or oblique alveolar bone loss can be a sign of a *split tooth*.

RULES OF THUMB:
- Where no reason can be seen for pulpal or periapical signs or symptoms, the likelihood that the tooth is cracked increases proportionally with the

(A)

(B)

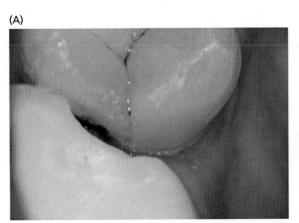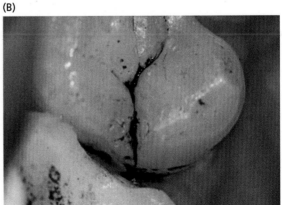

Fig. 13-13 The use of dyes (e.g. Methylene Blue or vegetable dyes) can help to identify the presence of an otherwise difficult-to-see crack. While a crack is barely visible in the distal marginal ridge of this premolar (A) it is much easier to see when the crack is stained with Methylene Blue dye (B) (image courtesy of Dr Unni Krishnan).

(A)   (B)

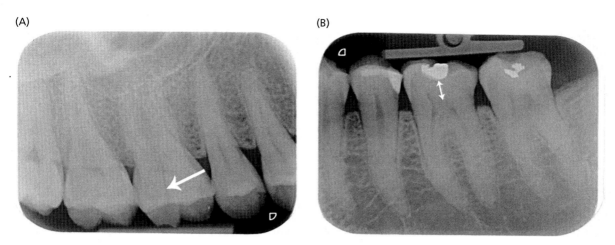

Fig. 13-14 (A) A symptomatic, unrestored maxillary molar tooth with acute pulpitis. A vertical crack is evident on the periapical radiograph (arrow). (B) A minimally restored symptomatic mandibular first molar tooth. The smaller the restoration and the greater distance between the restoration and the pulp (double arrow), the greater the chance the tooth has a deep mesiodistal crack (radiographs courtesy of Dr Unni Krishnan).

(A)   (B)

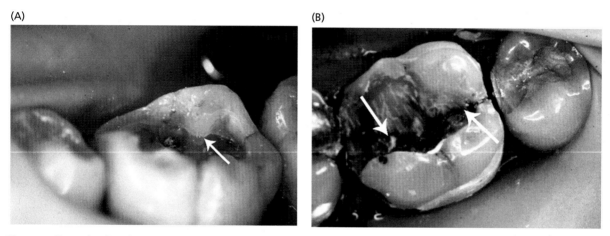

Fig. 13-15 Example of cracks in teeth. (A) A cracked cusp. Note the change in color of the tooth structure at the pulpo-axial line angle (arrow) and the crack across the distal marginal ridge. (B) A cracked tooth. Note the stained line extending mesiodistally across the pulpal floor (arrows).

increasing thickness of dentin present between the restoration and the pulp (or the shallower the restoration). A crack extending into the pulp chamber is most likely the cause of pulpitis or pulp necrosis.

• The smaller the restoration in a tooth with a crack, the deeper and more unfavorable the crack will be. All cracks in unrestored teeth are unfavorable, unless the patient has suffered indirect trauma, where the maxillary and mandibular teeth have been forcibly brought into contact.

Other signs and symptoms of a crack

There are situations where examination of a symptomatic tooth does not reveal any obvious reason for pulpal pathosis. In considering these cases, it is helpful to reflect on *what might have changed in the tooth that has caused it to become symptomatic.* When symptoms develop in a tooth that appears reasonably intact and has been adequately restored for many years, a crack has to be suspected.[109]

Ask: *"What has changed to make this previously non-painful tooth now exhibit symptoms?"*

3. Crack investigation

To confirm that a crack is present, it is necessary to remove the entire restoration and thoroughly cleanse the underlying dentinal surface. Close investigation of remaining tooth structure under magnification and bright light (fiber-optic) is essential to visualize most cracks in teeth. Smoothing out sharp angles with a large round bur and the use of a bright (fiber-optic) light is helpful.

A marked color change at the pulpo-axial line angle is an indication that the tooth is cracked. Other cracks appear as lines in the tooth structure. They may be clear or stained (Fig. 13-15). *Some cracks are not immediately visible and only become apparent once the surface of the dentin dries out.* The edges of some cracks may then appear frosted. In cuspal cracks, the more frosted the margin of the crack appears, the thinner the cracked segment and the more favorable the prognosis of the crack.

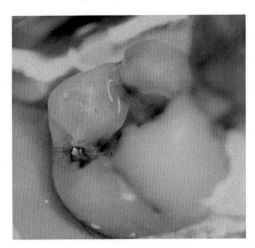

Fig. 13-16 Cracks involving the two lingual cusps of a second molar are clearly seen when the cavity preparation is filled with water; light refraction makes the cracks easier to see.

When examining a crack, the tooth should be either *dry or wet, but not damp*. When the tooth is wet, the refraction of light magnifies the crack, making it more visible (Fig. 13-16). It is difficult to see a crack when the dentinal surface is *damp*. Scattering and reflection of light from the damp surface make the crack difficult to visualize. Isolation of the tooth with a rubber dam greatly assists in the visualization of the crack.

4. Treatment planning

Once the nature and location of a crack are determined, the treatment plan will depend on the *type of fracture* present, *the amount of remaining tooth* structure, probing depths and the *symptoms* the patient is experiencing. A simple treatment classification for cracked teeth involves consideration of these factors.

Type of crack

From a treatment perspective, cracks can be classified as being favorable or unfavorable cracks, or a split tooth:

Favorable cracks

A *cusp is cracked*. In a favorable crack, only a cusp (or cusps) is fractured. The pulp may or may not be involved (Figs 13-17 and 13-18).

Unfavorable cracks

The tooth itself is cracked. Unfavorable cracks (Fig. 13-19) occur across the roof of the pulp chamber, in the pulp chamber or in intact unrestored teeth. These cracks pass deeply into the tooth structure. The pulp space is likely to be involved (Fig. 13-19).

It is possible for teeth to have both favorable and unfavorable cracks (Fig. 13-20).

Split tooth

The tooth has completely split into two segments. A tooth is classified as split when it is no longer intact and there is independent mobility of both segments (Fig. 13-21).

Cracked teeth fracture in a "crown down" manner. Many authors include vertical root fractures in posterior teeth in discussions of cracked teeth. In anterior root-filled teeth, vertical root fractures often occur from the crown down towards the root apex. It is possible for a coronal crack in a molar tooth to progress through the tooth into the root to create a vertically fractured crown and root. This often occurs in a mesiodistal direction following the direction of the initial crack. Vertical root fractures in posterior teeth, on the other hand, progress in the direction from the apex towards the crown. They rarely progress into the crown of the tooth. Most occur in a bucco-lingual direction and involve the broader roots (the mesio-buccal roots of maxillary molars and mesial roots of mandibular molars). They result in mild to moderate pain and are invariably associated with radiographic or clinical evidence of vertical bone loss.[108] Most, but not all, vertical root fractures in posterior teeth are associated with root-filled teeth.[110,111]

Type of pain

A patient's symptoms are important when planning treatment. A cracked tooth can exhibit pulpal or periapical symptoms:

- *No pain*: crack is discovered during a restorative procedure.
- *Symptoms suggestive of reversible pulpitis*: sharp pain of momentary duration that occurs only when the tooth is stimulated.
- *Symptoms suggestive of irreversible pulpitis*: prolonged stimulation or unprovoked pulpal pain.
- *Periapical pathosis*: symptoms associated with apical periodontitis or apical abscess (includes asymptomatic teeth with non-vital pulps).

The simple treatment classification for cracked teeth below facilitates treatment planning decisions and takes into consideration the above factors:

- Favorable crack/no pain or reversible pulpitis
- Favorable crack/irreversible pulpitis (or an exposed pulp)
- Favorable crack/periapical pathosis
- Unfavorable crack/reversible pulpitis
- Unfavorable crack/irreversible pulpitis (or an exposed pulp)
- Unfavorable crack/periapical pathosis.

It is not the intent of this manual to discuss treatment options for cracked teeth in detail. There are, however, some basic principles that are common to most treatment protocals.

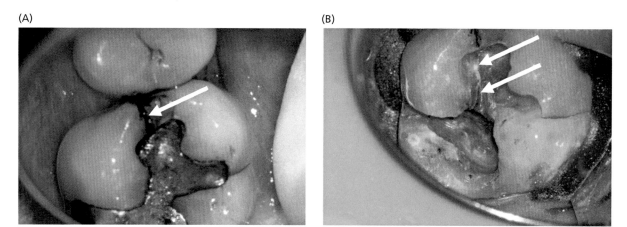

Fig. 13-17 Favorable (cuspal) crack. Note in the preoperative image (A) the difference in color between the buccal cusps and the mesiopalatal cusp, which is cracked. Staining shows the presence of a crack across the mesial marginal ridge (arrow). Removal of the restoration (B) reveals that the mesiopalatal cusp is cracked (arrows) (images courtesy of Dr Unni Krishnan).

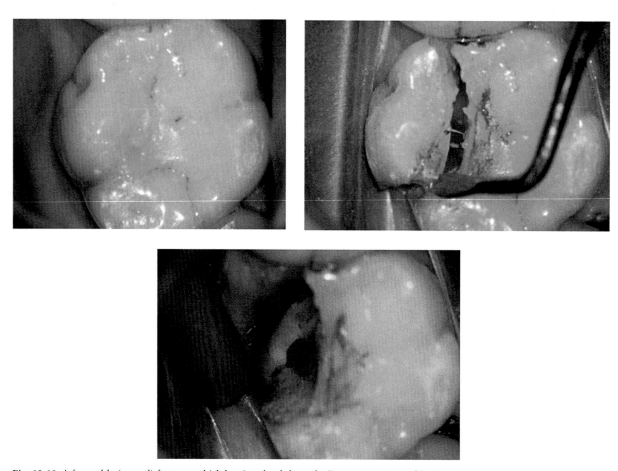

Fig. 13-18 A favorable (cuspal) fracture which has involved the pulp (images courtesy of Dr Unni Krishnan).

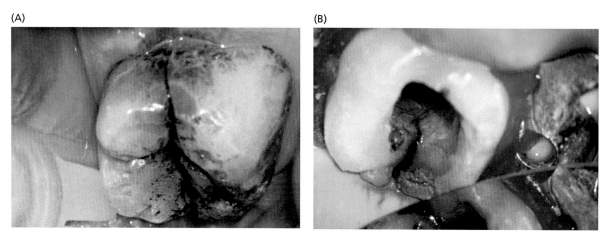

Fig. 13-19 Unfavorable cracks pass deeply into tooth structure. In (A), an unfavorable mesiodistal crack in an unrestored lower molar has been stained with Methylene Blue. In (B), an unfavorable crack can be seen passing into the pulp chamber.

(A)   (B)

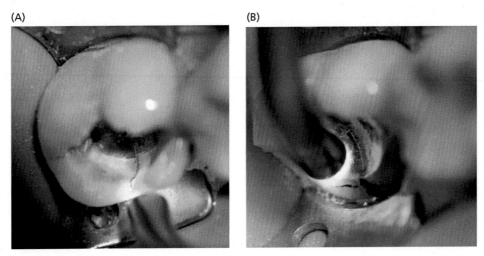

Fig. 13-20 A symptomatic tooth with two cracked lingual cusps. When the cusps were removed, a bucco-lingual unfavorable crack was also apparent.

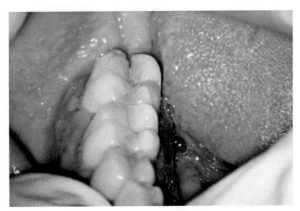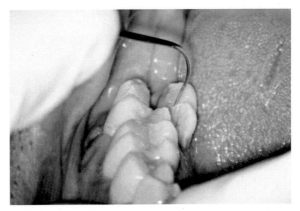

Fig. 13-21 A split tooth. A mesiodistal fracture has resulted in a complete separation of a lingual crown-root segment from the rest of the tooth (images courtesy of Dr Unni Krishnan).

Often teeth with cracks are not symptomatic, cracks being discovered when restorations are being replaced. Symptoms only present if the dentin is able to conduct a stimulus to the pulp. Thus, many teeth can be cracked but asymptomatic. For these teeth, conservative full cuspal coverage or no treatment may be the treatment of choice. Full coverage with composite resin restorations is sometimes an option, but occlusal modification to reduce the forces on the tooth is desirable before this is done.

Treating favorably cracked teeth

The treatment of *symptomatic favorably cracked* teeth is relatively straightforward, usually involving restoration after removal of the cracked cusp and treatment of any pulpal problems. Most cracked cusps separate at the level of the cemento-enamel junction. Those that do not are often associated with the larger (bulkier) cusps such as the palatal cusp of maxillary posterior teeth. An important factor to consider when treatment planning for favorable cracks is the amount of remaining tooth structure that is present. Successful restorative management is dependent on the amount of remaining supragingival tooth

structure. The prognosis is excellent, provided sufficient tooth structure remains.

Teeth can present with several cracked cusps. Teeth with multiple fractured cusps and intact pulps may require crown-lengthening procedures for restorative purposes or endodontic therapy. Endodontic treatment if required, is not compromised by the presence of a cuspal crack.

Current advances in composite resin materials and bonding techniques have allowed some of these favorable cracks to be treated more conservatively. This may be the first treatment of choice. However, only a few studies support bonding cracked cusps to the remaining tooth structure for the medium term.[112-114]

Treating unfavorably cracked teeth

There are few reliable long-term scientific data on treatment planning for teeth with unfavorable cracks.[112-116] The relationship you have with your patients and their expectations are as important in decision making as the state of the tooth. Anecdotally, many unfavorably cracked teeth without separation of the segments are treatable for the medium term, provided there are no associated probing depths or radiographic evidence of horizontal bone loss:

- Do not chase unfavorable cracks apically "to see where they go."
- Even with microscopy, it is not possible to see the full extent of unfavorable cracks. Thus, treatment decisions should not be made based on the *presumed depth of a crack*. In molar teeth the pulp chamber is centered on the cemento-enamel junction. Thus, it can be assumed that all unfavorable cracks communicate with the pulp chamber. Therefore, decisions on whether to treat should therefore be based on the presence or absence of bone loss and on the pulp status.
- If non-vital cracked teeth are to be treated endodontically and not restored immediately, *protect the tooth by banding and place the core material with the band in place.*
- Unfavorable cracked teeth that have deep periodontal probing defects are not candidates for conservative management.

Prevention better than a cure

When considering treatment planning for any unfavorably cracked tooth, it is well to consider that a crack is usually an indication of occlusal problems (Fig. 13-22), and/or where a tooth has been weakened by the placement of intra-coronal restorations.[117] Treatment of the cracked tooth without examining the occlusion is poor practice and not in the best interest of the patient. Thus, when restoring posterior teeth, particularly in patients with a history of fracturing cusps:

- Cover all weakened cusps.
- Cap isolated molar cusps.

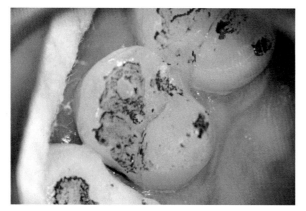

Fig. 13-22 A maxillary second premolar with a cracked palatal cusp. Examination of the occlusion is an important part of treatment planning for such a cracked tooth (image courtesy of Dr Unni Krishnan).

- Adjust the occlusion to remove excessive forces on cusps of posterior teeth.
- In cases showing severe occlusal wear, selectively narrow the occlusal table, thereby reducing the lateral forces on molar teeth.
- Identify and correct biting habits (e.g. chewing ice).
- Fabricate night guards where necessary, particularly if a patient has more than one cracked tooth or if there is evidence of a parafunctional habit.[118]

As with almost all treatment planning, a proper diagnosis is required before treatment is commenced. This is especially true for cracked teeth. Teeth that are cracked or give a previous history of being cracked need special management.

Questions to ask when considering a cracked tooth

Are any of your teeth sensitive to hot or cold?

Teeth with unexplained sensitivity to thermal changes should be suspected of being cracked until proven otherwise.

Do any of your teeth hurt when you bite on them?

A crack should be suspected in *vital* teeth that are sensitive to biting pressure.

What sort of pain do you feel?

Pain experienced in vital cracked teeth is usually very sharp and of short duration.

Does it hurt every time you bite?

A working cusp (e.g. buccal cusp of lower molar) is involved if it *hurts every time a patient bites* together.

A non-working cusp (e.g. lingual cusps of lower molars) is usually involved if it hurts "*only occasionally.*"

How long does it hurt after you drink something hot or cold, or if you bite on your teeth?

"Ouch and gone" is suggestive of reversible pulpitis, whereas "ouch and stays" is suggestive of irreversible pulpitis.

Does it hurt when you bite together or when you release the pressure?

Pain on release of pressure is a sign of a cracked tooth (or loose restoration or loose crown). A composite resin restoration which has debonded can have the same symptoms as a cracked tooth. To diagnose this, determine whether it is sensitive to pressure on the restoration alone, or when the pressure is applied to both the restoration and the adjacent tooth structure at the same time.

Do you remember anything happening when the pain started?

Some patients can remember the exact moment when a tooth cracked.

Chapter 14

Diagnosing Joint and Muscle Pains

Chris Moule and Iven Klineberg

Introduction

Pain arising from temporomandibular joint (TMJ) and the masticatory muscles is the most common non-odontogenic source of orofacial pain.[119] Thus, in diagnosis, consideration must be given to the possibility of pain arising from these structures. Diagnosis can be complicated by the fact that pain from muscles can be referred to the teeth and mimic toothache. Conversely, pain from teeth can be referred to muscles.

Patients often insist that they have toothache when in fact the pain is arising from a joint or muscle. Demonstration physically of muscular tenderness and the use of selective dental anesthesia can differentiate between the two types of pain. Without obvious infection, dental pathosis does not produce tenderness to palpation on the side of the face. Dental pain is also not relieved by the application of heat to the side of the face, whereas heat can relieve muscle pain. Of note is that muscle tenderness can develop from a patient's adaptive response to pain from another source or cause, and then it becomes the patient's major complaint.

In addition to screening and targeted questioning, a careful assessment of the mobility of the TMJ and palpation of the muscles of the head and neck are necessary. Palpation of the TMJ is undertaken by locating the joint just anterior to the tragus of the ear and pressing on it in closed and open positions and during dynamic opening or closing. Palpation of the posterior area of the lateral pole can be achieved by inserting the small finger into the ear and pressing on the anterior wall. Tenderness of the joint to palpation and pain on opening confirm a joint problem.

Localized hypersensitive bands of muscle fibers, *termed trigger points,* can develop within a muscle. Palpation of these can initiate referred pain to other sites. A note should be made of pain that is felt (by palpation) or relieved (by massage) at sites other than the one being stimulated. Although pain is produced at a site distant from the stimulated trigger point, there are no confirmatory signs of a problem at the site of referred pain. Sites for referred pain (site of the pain) from musculature (source of the pain) in the orofacial region (Figs 14-1 to 14-7) have been described in the literature.[120] Specific to the diagnosis of orofacial pain are referral patterns described for the following muscles:

Masseter

The superficial superior portion of the muscle can refer pain to maxillary molar teeth, whereas the superficial mid-belly portion can refer pain to the mandibular molar teeth. The superior part of the deep layer can refer pain to the TMJ.

Temporalis

Trigger points in the anterior, middle and posterior bodies of the muscle can refer pain to maxillary incisors, maxillary premolars and maxillary molars, respectively.

Digastric

The anterior belly can refer pain to the mandibular central incisor teeth and the posterior belly to the mastoid process.

Sternocleidomastoid (SCM)

The superficial sternal body of the SCM refers pain into the region of the TMJ and above the eyebrow. Pain referral should be suspected if the joint is not painful to palpation. The deep clavicular body of the muscle can refer to its post-auricular attachment and frontally above the eye. Headaches situated above

Diagnosing Dental and Orofacial Pain: A Clinical Manual, First Edition. Edited by Alex J. Moule and M. Lamar Hicks.

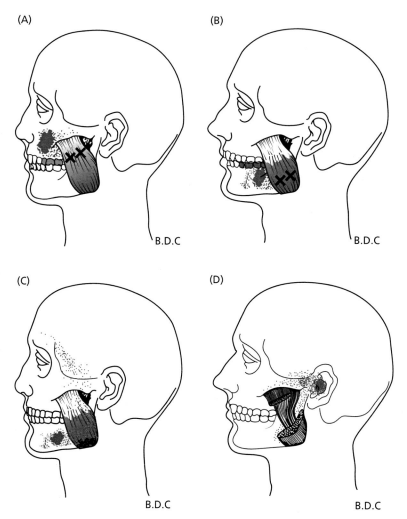

Fig. 14-1 The masseter muscle can refer pain (red) to the head and orofacial region, principally to the posterior teeth and infraorbital areas. Trigger points are marked as X. Referral pattern from the trigger point is dotted (from Simons, D.G., Travell, J.G. and Simons, L.S.[120], with permission).

the eye are commonly referred pain from the deep clavicular body or from the occipitofrontalis muscle.

Pterygoids

The *medial pterygoid muscle* can refer pain to the region of the TMJ.

The *lateral pterygoid muscle* can refer pain (red) to the head and orofacial region, principally to the zygomatic area and the TMJ.

Trapezius

The upper part of the muscle can refer pain to the lower border to the angle of the mandible, into the temporal area as well as occipitally and into the mastoid process.

Temporomandibular disorder

Temporomandibular disorder (TMD) is a general term reflecting dysfunction of the masticatory system. There are several subtypes, each with implications for treatment. Diagnosing TMD is complicated

because signs of joint disturbances can occur with or without demonstrable pain. Nevertheless, temporomandibular conditions usually present with consistent diagnostic signs and symptoms. This chapter is designed to help practitioners identify those signs and symptoms, which in turn will aid in more precisely selecting treatment modalities.

Pain from TMD typically originates from the masticatory muscles, the TMJ or chronic neuropathic mechanisms in response to these conditions. Previous classifications of TMD were based on anatomical models. However, in this manual the newer Diagnostic Criteria for TMD (DC-TMD) classification, which is based on a bio-psychosocial model, will be used.[121] In this bio-psychosocial model, pain is described with reference to two axes. Axis I refers to the physical assessment of the pain condition. Axis II refers to the psychosocial status and pain-related disability. With respect to joint and muscle pain:

- Axis I relates to the physical signs and symptoms of the disorder, and has two foundations: the source of the joint and muscle pain, and the

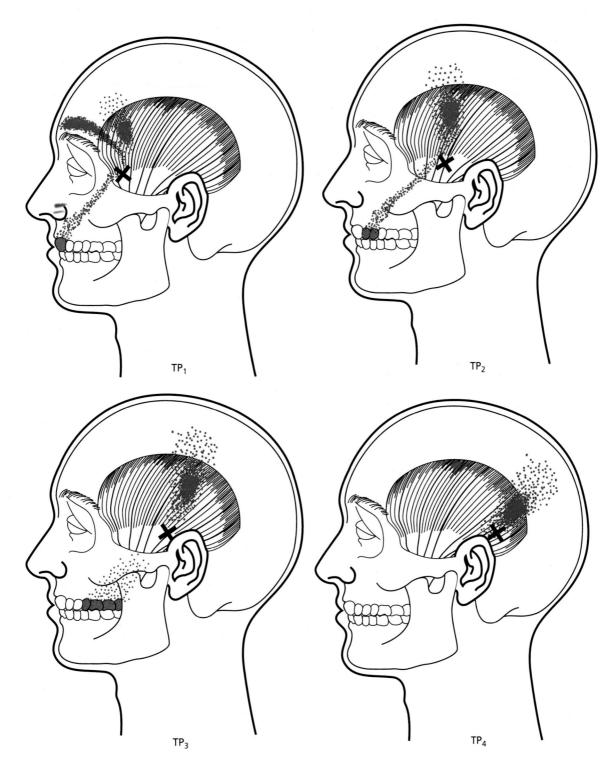

TP₁

TP₂

TP₃

TP₄

Fig. 14-2 The temporalis muscle can refer pain (red) to the head and orofacial region, principally to the maxillary teeth and temporal areas. Trigger points are marked as X. Referral pattern from the trigger point is dotted (from Simons, D.G., Travell, J.G. and Simons, L.S.[120], with permission).

presence (or absence) of an associated structural abnormality within the joint itself.

• Axis II relates to the psychosocial impact of the TMD condition.

It is outside the scope of this manual to discuss specific treatment modalities for TMJ conditions or discuss the psychosocial impacts of TMD. Excellent texts are available that describe both aspects of TMD.[122,123] The focus is placed first on the recognition of the physical signs and symptoms of symptomatic temporomandibular conditions, and second on the diagnosis of TMD. The physical diagnosis of temporomandibular disorders (Axis I) is based on:

a. the classification of the source of the patient's pain, and

b. the structural abnormality that may exist within the temporomandibular joint.

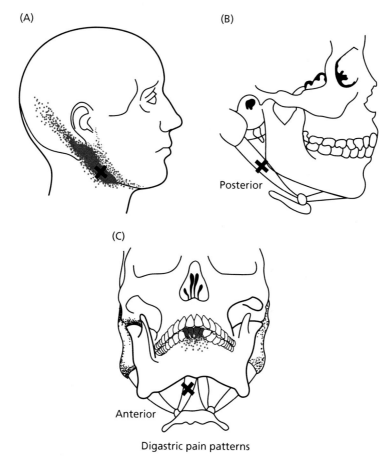

Fig. 14-3 The digastric muscle can refer pain (red) to the head and orofacial region, principally to the lower anterior teeth and posterior auricular areas. Trigger points are marked as X. Referral pattern from the trigger point is dotted (from Simons, D.G., Travell, J.G. and Simons, L.S.[120], with permission).

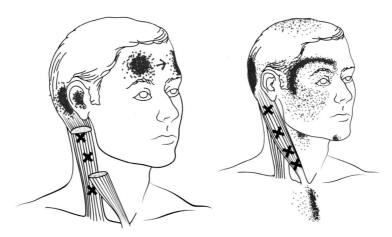

Fig. 14-4 The sternocleidomastoid muscle can refer pain (red) to the head and orofacial region, principally to the posterior auricular and peri-orbital regions. Trigger points are marked as X. Referral pattern from the trigger point is dotted (from Simons, D.G., Travell, J.G. and Simons, L.S.[120], with permission).

Temporomandibular disorders associated with pain

Temporomandibular disorders associated with pain are classified by the DC-TMD as:

1. Masticatory muscle disorders
2. Arthralgia (inflammation within the joint capsule)
3. Headache associated with TMD.

TMD may be associated with structural anomalies in the joint. The diagnostic criteria for the most common subtypes of structural abnormalities within the joint (*intra-articular temporomandibular disorders*) are:

1. Disc displacement with reduction
2. Disc displacement with reduction with intermittent locking

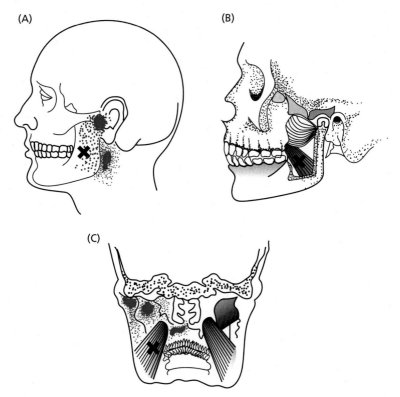

Fig. 14-5 Referral patterns for the medial pterygoid are illustrated in red. Trigger points are marked as X. Referral pattern from the trigger point is dotted (from Simons, D.G., Travell, J.G. and Simons, L.S.[120], with permission).

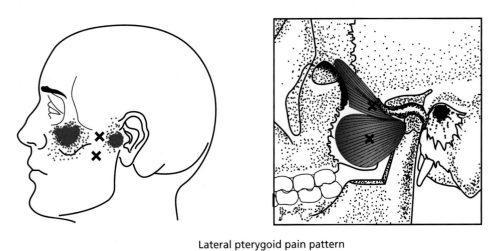

Lateral pterygoid pain pattern

Fig. 14-6 Referral patterns for the lateral pterygoid are illustrated in red. Trigger points are marked as X. Referral pattern from the trigger point is dotted (from Simons, D.G., Travell, J.G. and Simons, L.S.[120], with permission).

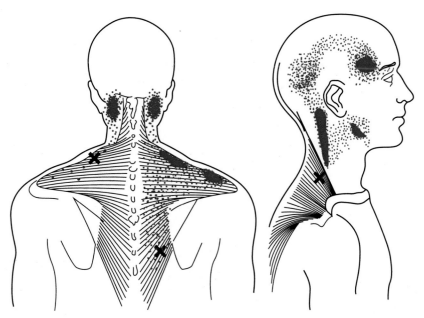

Fig. 14-7 Referral patterns for the trapezius muscle are illustrated in red. Trigger points are marked as X. Referral pattern from the trigger point is dotted (from Simons, D.G., Travell, J.G. and Simons, L.S.[120], with permission).

3. Disc displacement without reduction with limited opening
4. Disc displacement without reduction without limited opening
5. Degenerative joint disease
6. Subluxation.

It is important to consider that:

• One patient can present with a combination of *intra-articular temporomandibular disorders*.
• The treatment for each condition may be different.
• Each of three subtypes associated with pain may occur in relation to an intra-articular disorder or independently.
• Intra-articular disorders may occur *without* pain.

Jaw and muscle pain associated with TMD may also be classified as acute or chronic.

Acute jaw and muscle pains have an obvious cause and are of short duration. The pain may occur due to extreme wide opening with yawning, restoration of posterior teeth or extraction, biting on a hard object, or impact trauma such as a blow or fall. In each case, the cause is obvious to the patient and the clinician.

Chronic jaw and muscle pains do not have an obvious cause, especially where pain has been present for some months. Pain that has been present for some time may develop a neuropathic basis, which is more challenging to understand, diagnose and manage.[124,125] Chronic pain nevertheless is generally described as *always present* and may become severe. It is characterized by periods of exacerbation and remission. The constant chronic pain can resolve without apparent reason, and then reoccur without apparent cause. It is associated with elevated levels of stress resulting in increase in anxiety, somatization and often depression.

Masticatory muscle pain

The most common cause of non-odontogenic orofacial pain is masticatory muscle pain.[119] It is typically felt locally in the region of the affected muscles, but may be referred to the temple, cheek, neck or submandibular regions. Pain may be experienced when the muscle is active or stretched. Palpation of the muscle may reveal trigger points, which may refer pain to a distant site. Patients with muscle dysfunction commonly state that they experience pain *after* they eat.

Muscle pain has a dull ache quality, which may be constant or fluctuate in intensity. An episode of this type of pain may be present for a long time. A patient is likely to point to the region overlying the muscles of mastication or to sites of referral: typically the temple (temporalis muscle) or the cheek (masseter muscle). A description of a location deep within the cheek is suggestive of lateral pterygoid muscle involvement.

Pressing on affected muscles may elicit:

• Localized pain (*localized myalgia*)
• Pain that extends throughout the muscle (*myofascial pain without referral*)
• Pain that refers to other parts of the head and neck (*myofascial pain with referral*).

Muscle pain associated with trigger points often leads to pain referred into the head and neck. Similarly, sites in the neck can refer pain to masticatory muscles.[120] Analgesics often relieve the pain, but the relief may be brief. Antibiotics do not relieve the pain.

Confirmatory tests for jaw muscle pain

• Muscle pain is likely when palpation of superficial jaw and cervical musculature produces tenderness.
• Muscle pain is confirmed if palpation of muscles causes referred pain.
• A positive response to local treatment measures (e.g. moist heat) or a failure of local dental anesthesia to eliminate the pain helps differentiate jaw muscle pain from dental and other pains.

Treatment considerations for jaw muscle pain

• Application of moist heat will relieve acute muscle pain.
• Careful infiltration injection with an anesthetic solution without vasoconstrictor into a trigger point will relieve the pain.[126]
• While analgesics may have a limited effect in pain relief, muscle relaxants are more effective; however, their long-term use is contraindicated.
• Screening radiography is indicated to rule out dental or other pathosis. The treatment of chronic jaw muscle pain requires a thorough diagnostic work-up of the TMD condition, including a detailed clinical examination and imaging. Relaxation and stress management therapies can be considered.

Arthralgia

The term arthralgia refers to pain caused by *inflammation within the joint capsule*.[119] It is characterized by tenderness to palpation of the lateral pole of the condyle or pain in the joint with wide opening. This can be caused by trauma or any intra-articular disorder including disc displacements and arthritis.

Pain may be experienced in the region of the joint or in muscles associated with jaw movement. TMJ pain is usually described as *in front of the ear*, but may be felt in the ear. The pain tends to be more localized than muscle pain. Patients typically present with restriction in jaw movement, pain on jaw movement or joint sounds.

Confirmatory tests for arthralgia

Tenderness in the joint to palpation and pain with jaw movement are pathognomonic for temporomandibular conditions. Joint palpation is carried out in closed, opening and open positions.

Treatment considerations for arthralgia

Acute management of arthralgia involves jaw rest, anti-inflammatory medication and removal of causative factors, followed by a full assessment of the TMD condition.

Apart from initial local measures, treatment of chronic arthralgia requires complete clinical and radiographic examination and an accurate diagnosis before definitive treatment planning. Where pain has been present for some time, does not respond to initial treatment and has developed a neuropathic basis, psychosocial impacts require assessment. Medication, pain management, and relaxation and stress management therapies may need to be incorporated into the treatment.

Headaches associated with TMD

Headaches, usually tension type, with a *bilateral* dull pain character may be experienced secondary to temporomandibular disorders. Trigger points are characteristic of myofascial pain. Palpation of trigger points in the temporalis muscle (or other affected musculature) will reproduce or exacerbate the headache.

Although uncommon, temporomandibular conditions can be triggers for migraine-type headaches. Classic migraine symptoms include nausea and photosensitivity in conjunction with severe throbbing headaches. Although migraines are believed to be of neurovascular origin, many triggers have been reported, including temporomandibular pain.[122]

Diagnosing TMD

Contrary to popular belief, temporomandibular conditions usually present with consistent diagnostic symptoms. The following questions are designed to assist in identifying these signs and symptoms and confirm that a TMD condition exists. Precise treatment modalities can then be chosen based on the presence of symptoms and the intra-articular diagnoses in TMD determined by imaging and clinical examination.

Do you feel pain when opening your mouth?

Pain with jaw movement is pathognomonic for a temporomandibular condition. Pain is experienced in the joint or in muscles associated with jaw movement.

Where do you feel the pain?

Pain is usually described as being *in front of the ear*, but may also be felt *in the ear*. Location can help to determine the source, but consideration should be given to pain referral pathways. An absence of signs of inflammation in the ear helps to confirm a joint involvement.

Do you have difficulty opening your mouth or do you feel that your opening is restricted?

Patients with TMD often have restricted jaw opening. It is either a physical restriction, where the patient cannot force the jaw to open further, or a self-imposed limit to opening to minimize pain.

Does your jaw become stuck or locked, or go out of position?

Restricted opening may be caused by an intracapsular disorder, typically presenting as a closed lock, where a patient cannot open beyond 20–25 mm. This may be consistent or intermittent, depending upon the anatomical cause. Patients can develop a lateral deviated path of opening to avoid or overcome a restriction.

A *corrected deviation* occurs when the opening path deviates and then returns to the midline.

An *uncorrected deviation* occurs when the deviation persists through a full range of opening.

Do you have pain or difficulty when chewing, talking or using your jaws?

Pain with function may indicate inflammation within the joint capsule secondary to an intracapsular disorder or arthritis, or *muscle fatigue* in the presence of myofascial pain.

Do you have any noises in the jaw joints?

Jaw joints noises typically fall into two categories:

- *Clicking* is suggestive of an intracapsular disorder. In the absence of pain it is of little consequence. It is caused by a rapid movement of the articular disc with jaw opening and is typical of a disc displacement with reduction.
- *Crepitus* (a grinding sound) follows degenerative changes and is usually associated with perforation of the interarticular disc. It is caused by the articular surface of the condyle and glenoid fossa rubbing together with jaw movement. Patients may describe a *sandy* feeling. Crepitus is usually found either in disc displacements without reduction or in arthritis. In the absence of pain, crepitus is accepted as a variation of normal and does not usually require intervention.

Do your jaws frequently feel stiff, tight or tired?

This is typical of myofascial pain secondary to awake or sleep bruxism. Pain in the morning is suggestive of sleep bruxism. Pain increasing throughout the day is suggestive of daytime clenching.

Do you have frequent headaches, neckaches or toothaches?

TMD is characterized by periods of exacerbation and remission. Pain referral and persistent pain are common with chronic conditions. Multiple toothaches are not a characteristic of dental pain, and prolonged pain is rare.

Have you had a recent injury to your head, neck or jaw?

Temporomandibular conditions are usually caused by micro- or macro-trauma.

Macro-trauma describes a sudden, one-time traumatic incident causing physical damage to the joint or muscles.

Micro-trauma describes smaller injuries over a period of time, with the combined effect leading to physical symptoms (e.g. micro-trauma in nocturnal bruxism).

Are you aware of any recent changes in your bite?

A sudden change in the occlusion can be related to an acute disc displacement or a muscle spasm. Longer-term changes may be due to remodeling associated with arthritis.

When did the pain in your joint start?

The patient may describe a precipitating factor in an acute arthralgia scenario.

Intra-articular diagnoses in TMD

As stated above, treatment options for TMD have to take into consideration not only the disorders that cause pain, but also intra-articular disorders.[121] Intra-articular diagnoses are made in addition to the consideration of pain:

Disc displacement with reduction describes a click where there is no restriction in jaw opening. The displaced meniscus is recaptured as the jaw opens.

Disc displacement with reduction with intermittent locking occurs when a displaced meniscus prevents translation of the condyle by not reducing with jaw opening. A deviated path of opening often develops to avoid the obstruction in the affected joint.

Disc displacement without reduction with limited opening occurs when a displaced meniscus is not recaptured during the full range of jaw movement. Typically this will initially result in limitation in jaw movement and a closed lock condition. As the joint remodels, the limitation in movement may be overcome, but the disc remains located anterior to the condyle and is not recaptured with jaw opening.

Degenerative joint disease is characterized by joint remodeling and crepitus. It may occur with a general arthritis condition such as osteoarthritis or rheumatoid arthritis. Alternatively, it may reflect an ongoing remodeling procedure following an intracapsular disorder and be localized to the temporomandibular joint.[127]

Subluxation refers to locking of the jaw in the open-mouth position. It occurs when the condyle translates beyond the eminence and the articular disc prevents posterior translation. The patient will learn a technique for overcoming the obstruction and typically will self-restrict opening to avoid the open-lock condition.

Confirmation of intra-articular diagnosis (clinical examination)

Confirmation of the intra-articular diagnosis is made clinically and by imaging. The clinical examination involves observation of jaw movements and the effects of manipulation on the joint.

Deviation on opening occurs when one joint has reduced movement (translation-rotation), causing the mandible to deviate to the affected side.

Restricted opening may occur with joint or muscle dysfunction. The customary jaw opening is within the range of 40 to 60 mm, with males generally having wider jaw opening than females. Jaw opening of less than 30 mm indicates significant restriction. Muscle-based limitation may often be managed with home care. Joint-based dysfunction may be caused by disc displacement, fibrous adhesions within the joint or a reduced synovial fluid volume that limits joint mobility.

Clicking occurs as transient interruptions of disc movement associated with condyle movement. A click which has been present for a short time is more readily managed, while a longer duration suggests anatomical changes to the disc that are likely to persist. When a *click is eliminated with jaw protrusion*, it indicates a more favorable relationship between the disc and condyle, suggesting that conservative management with jaw exercises may reduce or eliminate the click.

Manipulation and provocation testing are designed to distract the affected condyle to allow the disc to assume a more favorable relationship with the condyle. This may be achieved by placing the forefingers (patient upright) or thumbs (patient supine) over the mandibular posterior teeth and pressing down to distract the condyles followed by moving the jaw forward. Manipulation often leads to an elimination of a click. But to maintain this relationship, the forward jaw and condyle position needs to be maintained to consolidate the disc relocation. This is usually achieved with protrusive jaw exercises or a repositioning appliance that is progressively modified to return the jaw to its original dental relationship.

Confirmation of intra-articular diagnosis (imaging)

Imaging may be indicated following a preliminary diagnosis based on history and clinical examination. The definitive imaging for intra-articular conditions is MRI, which differentiates hard and soft tissue detail. In addition, dynamic MRI can be used to image disc-to-condyle relationships with open-close movements. This allows clarification of the disc displacement with or without reduction (Fig. 14-8).

Where degenerative joint disease is present, a cone beam computed tomography (CBCT) scan can be used to show articular remodeling. Typical signs of this are (Fig. 14-9):

- *Flattening* of the articular surface of the condyle
- *Lipping or osteophyte formation*, which is seen radiographically as a spur from the condylar head
- *Subcondylar cyst formation*, which appears as isolated radiolucencies below the articular surface of

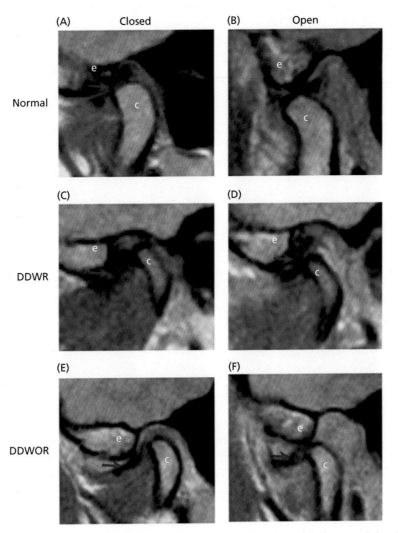

Fig. 14-8 Magnetic resonance imaging (MRI) images of the temporomandibular joint. (A) In the normal closed position, the disc (arrow) is positioned between the condyle and the articular eminence. (B) In the normal open position, the disc remains between the condyle and the eminence. (C) In the DDWR closed position, the disc is anteriorly displaced. (D) In the DDWR open position, the disc reduces into position between the condyle and the eminence. (E) In the DDWOR closed position, the disc is displaced anteriorly. (F) In the DDRWOD opening position, the disc remains displaced anteriorly throughout the range of movement. DDWR, disc displacement with reduction; DDWOR, disc displacement without reduction.

the condylar head with a disruption in the cortical border of the condylar head
- *Surface erosion*: Irregularities that develop on the condylar surface due to degenerative joint disease.

A. Normal appearance of a condylar head showing little evidence of degenerative change. While there is a large variation in the normal appearance of a mandibular condyle, most are convex in their superior outline with an intact cortical border.
B. There is marked flattening of the condylar head (arrowed) indicating significant resorption has occurred.
C. Subcondylar cyst formation (yellow arrow) and obliteration of the joint space (red arrow) in a severe degenerative joint condition.
D. The articular surface appears thin and eroded in this image (arrowed). Narrowing of the joint space and erosion of the condylar surface are indications of arthritic changes.

E. Lipping of the condylar head (arrowed) seen as a projection from the condylar surface due to the growth of an osteophyte is observed in this cross-sectional image.
F. Medial displacement of the condylar head secondary to a displaced fracture with healing in the displaced position (arrowed).

Treatment considerations for TMD

Depending on the diagnosis, treatment of TMD can be simple or very complex.[122] A low-tech, high-prudence approach has been advised with an emphasis on conservative, reversible therapies.[128] Treatment ranges from simple local measures, involving jaw rest, moist heat and analgesic medication, to complex splint therapy, pain management therapies and rarely surgery. Psychological assessment and medication may be required when there are psychosocial factors identified in chronic TMD. Only after an accurate

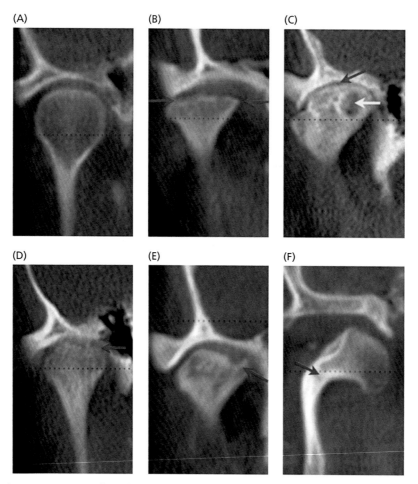

Fig. 14-9 CBCT imaging – cross-sections through condylar heads showing some morphological and radiological variations that can occur during remodeling, degenerative changes and disease processes.

diagnosis is made should definitive treatment be planned and carried out. It is therefore necessary to establish:

- that a temporomandibular condition exists and to differentiate it from other diagnoses.
- which of the subtypes of temporomandibular disorders associated with pain are present (muscle pain, arthralgia or headache associated with TMD).[121]
- whether the condition is acute or chronic.
- an accurate intra-articular diagnosis on which to base treatment planning.[121]
- whether psychosocial and neuropathic factors, including anxiety, somatization and depression, are compounding factors.[121]

Chapter 15

Diagnosing Pain Referral from Neck and Shoulders

Scott Cook and Alex J. Moule

Pain referral from neck and shoulders

The musculature controlling stability and movement of the cervical spine and shoulder girdle has an intricate relationship with jaw function. The muscles of mastication and normal jaw function (including chewing, talking, swallowing and yawning) assume that the cervical spine, particularly the upper cervical spine, is in central alignment and has adequate range of motion. Dysfunction and restriction of movement through the cervical region can lead to dysfunction of jaw systems, as they no longer have a stable base from which to operate Additionally, dysfunction in the cervical spine can also cause regional pain, which can be referred to the head and jaw. A thorough examination of the regional musculoskeletal system should therefore be undertaken to help identify and manage concurrent regional pain of non-dental sources in the head and jaw.

Pain referral from muscles

Muscles that have been damaged or chronically overloaded can develop points of tenderness. In acute injuries, the pain tends to be localized and is related to the associated inflammatory conditions present. However, with chronic overloading, trigger points can develop. These present as hyper-irritable spots in the fascia surrounding the muscle and are associated with palpable nodules or tight bands within the muscle fiber. Trigger points can be present in people who are asymptomatic, so their relevance to presenting regional pain is dependent on what type of pain they create when palpated. A so-called *dormant trigger point* creates only local radiating pain when palpated and is indicative of local muscle dysfunction only. This may be relevant to treatment in context with the presenting condition, but is not a primary source of

pain. Palpation of an *active trigger point* that is *tender locally and creates referred pain* to the region in question is indicative that the primary source of the pain is distal to the site of the pain. Evaluation of trigger points requires the practitioner to be competent in palpating muscles and to be able to identify areas of localized tension or bundling. An uninflamed muscle has the same consistency throughout.

By applying pressure directly to the middle of the tense area the practitioner can monitor the patient's response, including local pain, local muscle twitching and pain withdrawal, and noting whether pain is referred to the zone of reference or remains localized. This can assist in differentiating site versus source of pain. Confirmation of whether the suspected muscle is a primary contributor to the presenting pain can be made by either provoking the distal site (the muscle trigger point), and assessing its response or whether provocation reproduces results in pain referral, or assessing whether nerve blocking of the distal structure abolishes the referred pain.

Common pain referral patterns for muscles of the head and neck which can produce orofacial pain have been described extensively.[129] From a cervicogenic pain perspective, the upper trapezius muscle is a major source of referral[130] and can refer pain to the angle and lower border of the mandible, and into the temporal and suboccipital region (Fig. 15-1).

The *sternocleidomastoid muscle* (SCM) can refer pain to the head and orofacial region, principally to the ear, the TMJ, and supraorbital and suboccipital areas. Therefore, pain referral should be suspected if *"joint pain"* is present but the TMJ is not painful to palpation. The deep clavicular body of the SCM muscle can refer pain to its post-auricular attachment and frontally above the eye. Headaches situated above the eye are commonly referred pain from the deep clavicular

Diagnosing Dental and Orofacial Pain: A Clinical Manual, First Edition. Edited by Alex J. Moule and M. Lamar Hicks.
© 2017 John Wiley & Sons, Ltd. Published 2017 by John Wiley & Sons, Ltd.
Companion website: www.wiley.com/go/moule/dental_and_orofacial_pain

body of the SCM or from the occipitofrontalis muscle (Fig. 15-2).

Patterns of pain of referral from the muscles of mastication are described in Chapter 14.

Cervicogenic disorders

Cervicogenic disorders can involve the muscle, facet joints, discs and vertebrae of the cervical spine and can result in a wide variety of symptoms.[131] These symptoms can include localized neck pain during static or dynamic activities, loss of functional range of motion, local and regional muscle tenderness and hyper-tonicity (muscle spasm or guarding). If the pathology is significant (e.g. from a prolapsed degenerative disc), neurogenic symptoms may present including referral of pain to the upper limbs, head and face, pins and needles and altered touch sensation. Patients can also present with a cervicogenic headache, which usually presents as a unilateral constant dull ache, situated at the back of the head, behind the eyes or in the temple: or less commonly, on top of the head, forehead or ear. Only occasionally does cervicogenic pain present bilaterally.

Patients with cervicogenic disorders commonly present with adaptive or compensatory muscle behavior or postures. This is usually an attempt to protect an injured or painful structure from further damage while maintaining function. Unfortunately, these adaptive changes often lead to further problems, as they can allow continuation of the habits or functions that may have been contributing to their original problem. Common observable adaptations include:

Postural changes

Forward head and elevated, rounded shoulder positions to help brace, protect or avoid pressure on irritated structures including disc derangements or inflamed facet joints (Fig. 15-3).

Tongue scalloping

Scalloping along the lateral border of the tongue occurs as a result of the tongue being thrust laterally against the mandibular teeth. While there are a number of possible causes of tongue scalloping, it occurs when a patient braces the jaw using the tongue as a postural prop for inefficient control by anterior neck muscles and is a sign of a cervicogenic problem. An association with sleep apnea has been shown (Fig. 15-4).[132]

Elevated hyoid position

This results from inappropriate tongue activation and overactive or unbalanced superior hyoid muscle function, which can occur due to upper cervical spine

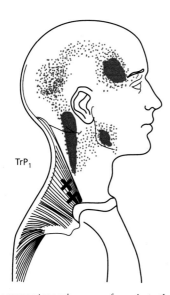

Fig. 15-1 The upper trapezius can refer pain to the angle and lower border of the mandible and into the temporal as well as suboccipitally. Trigger points are marked as X. Referral pattern from the trigger point is dotted (from Simons, D.G., Travell, J.G. and Simons, L.S., *Travell & Simons' Myofascial Pain and Dysfunction: The Trigger Point Manual*, 2nd edn. Baltimore: Williams and Wilkins, with permission).

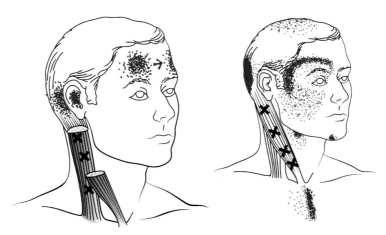

Fig. 15-2 The SCM can refer pain (red) to the head and orofacial region, principally to the ear, TMJ, supraorbital and suboccipital. Trigger points are marked with an X. Referral pattern from the trigger point is dotted (from Simons, D.G., Travell, J.G. and Simons. L.S. *Travell & Simons' Myofascial Pain and Dysfunction: the Trigger-point Manual*. 2nd edn. Baltimore: Williams and Wilkins, with permission).

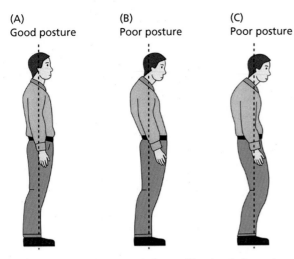

(A)
Good posture

(B)
Poor posture

(C)
Poor posture

Fig. 15-3 Observe the patient's forward head and elevated, rounded shoulder positions to help brace and protect inflamed structures.
(A) In good posture the patient has a good upright position.
(B) In poor posture the patient has a head-forward position and rounded shoulders. He has weak abdominal muscles and a sway back.
(C) In poor posture the patient has a head forward position and rounded shoulders. He also has a relatively flat back and compensates for this by bending his knees forwards.

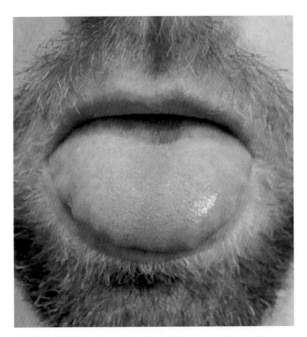

Fig. 15-4 Scalloping on the sides of the tongue due to the tongue being thrust laterally against the mandibular teeth as a postural prop to help stabilize the neck.

instability following trauma (e.g. whiplash injuries). Elevated hyoid positioning may manifest itself in a number of ways. Patients may have difficulty swallowing, clear their throat regularly and suffer speech changes. Patients who suffer whiplash injuries may also have eating difficulties.[133]

Temporomandibular disorders (TMDs)

The co-occurrence of TMDs and cervicogenic symptoms is well documented in the literature.[134–136] A cervicogenic origin should be considered if there is

pain in the region of the joint but no palpable tenderness in the joint. It is also possible to have multiple regional disorders contributing to a pain pattern, so it is important to systematically check all regional structures if referral from the neck or shoulders is suspected.

Common cervical spine disorders likely to present in a dental setting

A practitioner should be familiar with the pain referral patterns of nerves and musculature of the cervical spine, and be able to recognize that a cervicogenic problem is likely present. Dental practitioners also have a role to play in advising patients on the benefits of upper body exercises, stretching and attention to posture and regular exercise to reduce workplace muscle fatigue. While many practitioners will not have appropriate training to treat patients experiencing cervicogenic pain, recognition of symptoms and the origin of the problem is helpful in arranging referral.[137]

Cervicalgia

This refers to neck pain from any structure in general. It is often associated with SCM, upper trapezius and suboccipital tenderness. Patients with cervicalgia generally respond to a basic range of motion exercises and correction of posture.

Cervical strains and sprains

These often occur following trauma (e.g. whiplash injuries) affecting specific joint, muscle or disc structures. Treatment involves more specific management of underlying injuries.

Cervical osteoarthritis

Overloading of joint structures can result in inflammation and progressive degeneration of load-bearing structures. Treatment requires management to slow progression of the condition by first identifying and modifying causative factors (e.g. work posture). Cervical osteoarthritis can respond to targeted strength and range-of-motion exercises, despite poor appearance on radiographs.

Radiculopathy

Compression of nerve roots can cause sensorimotor deficit and/or pain, secondary to disc herniation, degenerative conditions or instability. These compressive injuries require specialist investigation including diagnostic imaging and possible neurosurgical review.

Examination of cervicogenic disorders

An examination of a patient who may be experiencing cervicogenic discomfort should include:

Posture assessment

Poor posture and overload of the cervical spine structures can result in acute inflammatory conditions and lead to long-term degenerative changes and chronic pain problems which can contribute to orofacial pain. Therefore, postural assessment should be conducted in all patients suspected of having cervicogenic pain or dysfunction, to determine whether there is any relationship between this and their orofacial pain.[138] This includes observing the patient in upright postures (sitting or standing), preferably in positions that are known to exacerbate their symptoms. Observations are made from in front, behind and from the side of the patient to best evaluate and visualize all aspects of their posture.

Neck and shoulder positions should be assessed for asymmetry from a frontal view. Signs of poor posture include subtle tilting of the head laterally or unilateral rotation, uneven shoulder elevation or depression, and asymmetry in muscle tone in the anterior neck muscles, including the SCM, scalenes and upper trapezius.

The upper back muscles, including the levator scapulae, middle and lower trapezius, and cervical extensor muscles, are better observed from behind. Asymmetry of scapular positions such as elevation, depression or rotation should be noted.

The extent of any forward head position and rounding of shoulders, as well as increased or decreased thoracic kyphosis (curvature), are best viewed from the side. Any asymmetry or shift from normal posture is a sign of potential compensatory muscle action or protective posturing for underlying cervical or regional (shoulder, upper back) dysfunction, and warrants investigation.

During observation of posture it may be possible to evaluate whether correction or changes in posture influence the patient's pain. While no immediate change in symptoms does not rule out the posture as contributory (postural load is a product of position and time), any immediate change in symptoms does confirm involvement of the structures and will require further management (postural correction advice) or referral for more comprehensive evaluation. For example, does correcting forward head posture reduce or increase suboccipital or headache pain?

Palpation

Palpation of the cervical region and surrounding structures is an important part of the physical examination and can help determine which structures may be contributing to regional pain, as well as conforming compensatory postural patterns. While more specific training and knowledge are required to ascertain specific structural diagnostics (such as identifying specific spinal segment or joint structure involvement), a broad overview of regional dysfunction and its possible contribution to orofacial pain can be gained through palpation of superficial muscle and joint structures, thus alerting the practitioner to the need for appropriate management or referral.

Common palpation points in the cervical spine include the upper trapezius, SCM and occipital extensor muscles. Tenderness or hypertonicity (over activity or unusual firmness) in these key anti-gravity muscles is a clear sign of overloading of the cervical region, as these muscles adapt and respond to sustained altered postural load to protect underlying neck structures. As previously mentioned, in trigger point referred pain, palpation of these overactive muscles can also reproduce distal pain, including headache and facial pain, and is a clear indicator of cervical muscle involvement in regional pain.

More specific palpation tests can be carried out by experienced clinicians trained in management of cervicogenic disorders to determine more exact structural injuries and their contribution to the presenting pain. These may include intersegmental examination of facet joint and disc structures to evaluate capsule or ligament injury at each level of the cervical spine, upper cervical ligament stability tests and regional sensitization tests, such as sub-occipital triangle palpation, and sustained segmental overpressure techniques.[139]

Suboccipital triangle palpation

Palpation of the upper cervical spine is a useful tool for determining the potential contribution of the spine to regional orofacial pain. Palpation with overpressure along the superior and inferior suboccipital margins is carried out within the area illustrated in Fig. 15-5, while gently extending the patient's neck (tipping the head backwards). While it is generally tender in this region, a sharp withdrawal response to palpation is a positive test result.

Movement tests

Evaluation of the cervical range of motion is an important part of examining the cervical spine, and it can be used to identify a pain source or functional range limitation and as a re-evaluation tool following treatment. Neck movements are examined for range of movement in flexion, extension, rotation and lateral flexion (Figs 15-6 and 15-7) (Table 15-1). As a general rule, the range of motion should be pain free and appear unrestricted and symmetrical, and movements should be smooth and well controlled. Any variation from this requires further expert examination.

As the upper cervical spine (C0–3) is commonly involved in referring pain to the orofacial region, differentiating and identifying upper neck restriction can be useful in determining whether a patient should be referred. A skilled clinician can assess this by stabilizing C3 manually from behind the patient, and asking the patient to repeat the movements. C0–1 and C1–2 joints are designed for movement and contribute to approximately half of the neck's available range. Disproportionate loss of upper cervical range (>50% loss of the entire range of motion of the neck) is indicative of a mechanical upper cervical dysfunction and requires further evaluation and treatment.

Radiographs

The finding of degenerative changes on imaging does not correlate with neck pain or disability.[140] Imaging of the cervical spine is mainly used to rule out gross discal lesions, nerve entrapments, fractures and other non-mechanical issues (e.g. tumors). Used as a tool with reference to other examination findings, radiography can help in diagnosis and management of patients, but must be considered in context of the presenting condition.

More specific evaluation of the relationship between the neck and jaw function can be performed on lateral transcranial views, and can be useful in confirming physical findings and guiding management. This analysis involves comparison of set joint angles and skeletal markers in upright posture compared to standardized ranges and helps identify deviation from normal positions which in turn helps direct treatment.

Treatment considerations

Treatment of cervicogenic pain problems is not normally within the scope of general practitioners. Recognition of a problem and appropriate referral to a relevant expert practitioner, familiar and experienced with these problems, are appropriate. Physical therapists (physiotherapists) and musculo-skeletal specialists are the most common referral points. It is important, however, to select from these specialists who are familiar with the complexities of managing associations between jaw joint pain, neck and shoulder problems and the presence of orofacial pain.[137]

If neck or shoulder involvement is suspected, appropriate referral to an experienced practitioner will either confirm or deny involvement of the musculature

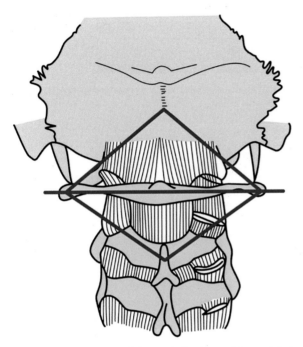

Fig. 15-5 Posterior view of the cervical spine and the occipital bone. The suboccipital region is drawn over the diagram in dark blue. Sensitivity to palpation of the upper cervical spine in this area is a strong indicator of a regional problem – occipital bone (ocher) and vertebrae (light blue).

(A)   (B)

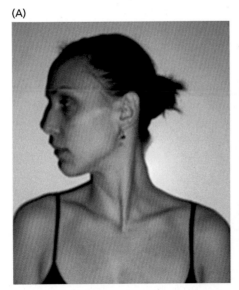 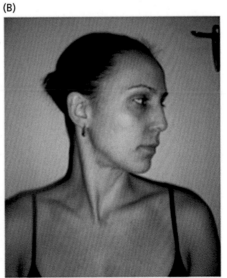

Fig. 15-6 Assessment of cervical spine rotation. In (A), the chin in alignment with the shoulder at a full 80-degree rotation range to the right, while (B) shows a restriction of movement to the left with the chin forward of the shoulder at end of available range.

(A)

(B)

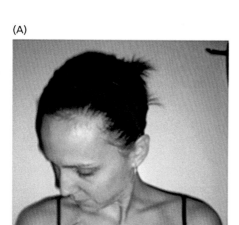
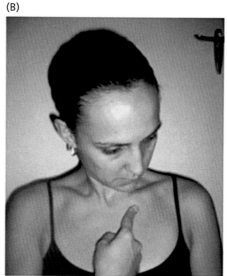

Fig. 15-7 Assessment of rotation in forward flexion, indicative of C0–2 segmental range of motion, which accounts for approximately 50% of the whole neck range. In (A), there is little restriction of movement as indicated by the chin alignment half-way across the clavicle. C0–2 segmental restriction is evident in (B), where chin alignment is only one-quarter across the clavicle.

Table 15-1 Direction of movements and expected ranges for flexion, extension, rotation and lateral extension. These measurements are used as a guide only, as range of movement varies greatly among individuals.

Flexion	Tipping head forwards	50–60 degrees
Extension	Tipping head backwards	55 degrees
Rotation	Turning head to side	80–90 degrees
Lateral flexion	Tipping head to side	45 degrees

in a patient's orofacial pain profile and confidently direct the next appropriate course of action. Some indications for referral are as follows:

- If neck pain immediately precedes the facial pain
- If jaw pain progresses to a temporal frontal or tension-type headache
- If neck movement makes the facial pain worse
- If there is significant movement restriction or postural deformity
- If the patient's neck becomes stiff or aggravated either from lying in the dental chair or after procedures
- If the pain has followed a previous whiplash-associated injury.

To avoid confusion over the required assessment of and treatment for the patient's orofacial pain problem, it is imperative also that a referring practitioner clearly communicates: 1) the reason for referral, 2) the presence of orofacial pain and 3) the treatment and examination that have already been undertaken. The treatment of chronic or referred orofacial pain requires a team effort. In addition to the written referral, clarification via a phone conversation in addition can facilitate the process.

Treatment hinges on a thorough cervicogenic assessment identifying the exact cervicogenic condition that is present. This ensures that treatment is focused on correcting the underlying disorder, rather than symptom relief. Depending on the case, treatment may include direct manual techniques such as joint mobilization, soft tissue massage and corrective exercise therapy. Other adjunctive modalities such as TENS, laser therapy, acupuncture or dry needling, and heat and cold therapy are also commonly used to assist in treatment, but are rarely the focus of long-term therapy; rather, they are temporary relieving modalities which assist with well-directed manual therapy.

Most importantly, the patient must be educated regarding their condition so they can effectively assist in their own management through understanding of aggravating and easing factors, and compliance with self-directed exercise and stretching strategies. Treatment can often take place over many months, so it is important to set reasonable expectations for the progress of successfully managing the pain from the outset of treatment to avoid the patient becoming frustrated with the process.

Useful questions if pain referral from neck and shoulder is suspected

Where is the main pain located?

Often patients will be aware of associated neck and shoulder muscle discomfort and can direct you to the muscles that are likely to be involved.

How and where does the pain start?

Neck or shoulder restriction or pain can often precede the onset of intermittent facial pain. For example, the patient will report feeling a painful neck restriction which then turns into jaw or other orofacial pain.

How would you describe the pain?

While it can vary in intensity, muscle pain is often described as a constant dull pain.

Do you usually get pain on both sides?

Cervicogenic headache usually occurs unilaterally. Associated shoulder discomfort is usually worse on one side.

Does anything make the pain worse?

Pain may be aggravated by activities including chewing and talking, or sustained postural tasks, such as computer work and uncomfortable work positions. It can usually be explained by sustained compromised muscle function or loading of compromised joint structures (i.e. mechanical loading). Other activities that may exacerbate neck and shoulder pain include slouching, excessive bending or twisting, or prolonged activities involving holding the arms outstretched.

Have you had a neck and shoulder injury or trauma?

A previous history of trauma can predispose a patient to neck pain. The elucidation of neck injury may identify a possible timeline of adaptation. Long adaptation periods increase the complexity of management.

Do you feel there might be an association between this injury and the pain you are having now?

While a patient's recall may not be accurate, a historical association between the current pain and a past event is helpful.

Can you have facial pain without neck pain or are the two areas painful together?

A cervicogenic problem is more likely if neck and face pain occur together.

Have you had a whiplash injury or a car accident?

Patients who have had an untreated whiplash injury can experience pain many years afterwards. The injury could have occurred many years prior to the appearance of neck and orofacial pain.

Do you have any difficulty swallowing?

Patients with neck injuries from a whiplash injury can complain of difficulties with eating and swallowing food.

Have you noticed any pain or restriction with neck or shoulder movements?

Other questions relating to function can include:

Can you turn your head freely from side to side?
Can you turn your head to reverse the car?
Can you hold your arms above your head comfortably?
Can you look up without discomfort?
Can you sit at the front of a movie cinema without discomfort?

Any restriction of movement is a sign of problems with the cervical spine. Restriction of movement or discomfort on movement can be due to either muscles or a structural problem in the spine. Patients with both orofacial pain and neck pain or restricted neck movement should be screened for cervicogenic causes.

Does your facial pain change with different neck or shoulder movements or with change in posture?

An association between neck movement and pain confirms a cervicogenic cause.

Have you had any treatment for a recurring neck pain?

A previous history of neck pain may suggest a cervicogenic cause for an orofacial pain problem. Most patients who have suffered neck pain are vulnerable to recurrence.

Chapter 16

Diagnosing Pain from the Sinuses

Unni Krishnan and Alex J. Moule

Introduction

The paranasal sinuses are four pairs of hollow air-filled cavities within the skull located on either side of the nose. They are called the maxillary, ethmoidal, frontal and sphenoidal sinuses (Fig. 16-1). They help reduce the weight of the skull, improve voice resonance and produce mucous which moisturizes the mucosal lining of the nasal cavity.

Classification of sinus pain

The general term, rhinosinusitis, which includes maxillary sinusitis, refers to a spectrum of disorders involving concurrent inflammation of the nasal cavity and paranasal sinuses. Inflammation in any of these can result in a variety of orofacial pain conditions. Rhinosinusitis can be classified as acute, recurrent, sub-acute or chronic.

Acute rhinosinusitis is an acute infection characterized by two or more signs and symptoms, one of which can be nasal obstruction, blockage, congestion or nasal discharge. These may be associated with facial pain, pressure, or a reduction in or loss of smell.[141] The term *acute sinusitis* is reserved for patients who have episodes lasting for up to four weeks:

- *Recurrent acute rhinosinusitis*: Patients who suffer four or more bouts of acute rhinosinusitis in a 12-month period are classified as having *recurrent acute rhinosinusitis*.
- *Subacute rhinosinusitis*: Rhinosinusitis lasting up to 12 weeks is classified as *sub-acute*.
- *Chronic rhinosinusitis*: This is more difficult to define due to the wide spectrum of clinical signs and symptoms and a lack of objective findings. It is generally defined as an infection producing nasal obstruction, blockage, congestion or discharge that persists for more than 12 weeks.[141]

Rhinosinusitis can also be classified according to signs and symptoms:[142]

- *Local*: Prominent symptoms include nasal congestion, obstruction and discharge, facial pain, facial fullness, headache and olfactory dysfunction.
- *Regional*: Symptoms include sore throat, dysphonia, cough, halitosis, bronchospasm and ear fullness and pain. Eustachian tube dysfunction and dental pain are present.
- *Systemic*: Symptoms include fatigue, malaise and fever. Anorexia can also occur.

Maxillary sinusitis presenting as toothache or facial pain

The maxillary sinus is the largest paranasal sinus. It communicates with the middle meatus of the nasal cavity through the ostium, which is highly innervated and the most sensitive of all nasal and paranasal structures.[143] Mucosal inflammation in or around the ostium contributes significantly to the pain experienced during an acute episode of sinusitis. Diseases involving the maxillary sinus are one of the most common causes of non-odontogenic dental pain.[143]

Pain arising from maxillary sinusitis can present in different ways:

1. Pain can be intense in the maxilla. There may be headache and *fullness* in the maxillary sinus, with exacerbations of pain during postural changes. Maxillary molar teeth may feel strange or *woody*. The patient may exhibit fever and malaise and complain of a post-nasal drip, which may produce a cough.
2. Pain can also present as a deep, prolonged, constant and unrelenting ache in the maxilla without any other obvious symptoms, which lasts for hours or days without treatment. The pain is probably due to mucosal edema (swelling)

Diagnosing Dental and Orofacial Pain: A Clinical Manual, First Edition. Edited by Alex J. Moule and M. Lamar Hicks.
© 2017 John Wiley & Sons, Ltd. Published 2017 by John Wiley & Sons, Ltd.
Companion website: www.wiley.com/go/moule/dental_and_orofacial_pain

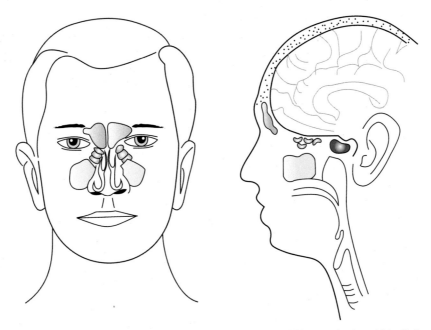

Fig. 16-1 The relative positions of the maxillary (beige), frontal (purple), ethmoid (blue) and sphenoid (red) sinuses are shown (adapted from http://www.cancer.gov/cancertopics/pdq/treatment/paranasalsinus/Patient/National Cancer Institute, National Institutes of Health, accessed 25 July 2015).

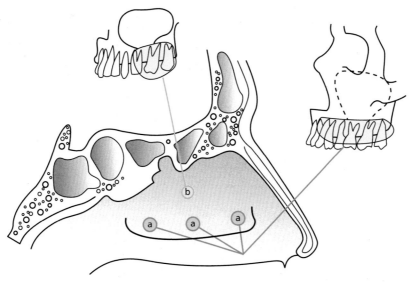

Fig. 16-2 Stimulation of the turbinates (a) can cause referred pain to all maxillary teeth. Stimulation of the ostium (b) can cause referred pain to maxillary molars (adapted from Wolff 1963).[145]

causing obstruction of the sensitive ostium. It is relieved by steam or medical inhalation therapy and decongestant nose drops.[144] In the absence of nasal symptoms, the diagnosis is confirmed retrospectively by observing the patient's response to the inhalation therapy and decongestants.

3. Several *vital* maxillary teeth may be sensitive to cold or percussion. Stimulation of the turbinates and the ostium can refer pain to maxillary molar teeth (Fig. 16-2) and to the face (Fig. 16-3).

4. In severe cases, maxillary molar teeth can become mobile and acutely painful, and the periodontal ligament can become widened (Fig. 16-4).

Patients with chronic rhinosinusitis may present with a history of pain present on waking; it no pain once they arise, but pain again later in the day. A common finding is severe congestion in the forehead (between the eyes) and in the maxilla (facial congestion).[146]

Maxillary sinusitis of dental origin

Maxillary sinusitis can result from an odontogenic infection, which invariably occurs unilaterally. Unilateral, recalcitrant rhinosinusitis with a foul odor is strongly suggestive of an odontogenic origin.[147] It is responsible for 70% of unilateral chronic paranasal sinusitis. If there is thickening of the sinus mucosa and the sinus cavity is filled with fluid up to two-thirds of its volume, there is an 86% chance that

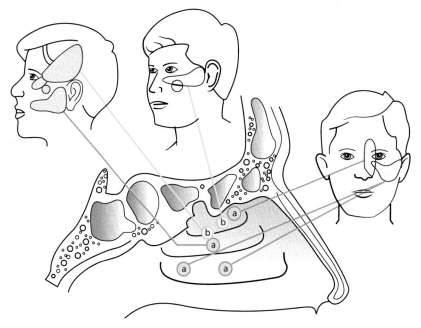

Fig. 16-3 Stimulation of the turbinates (a) can cause referred pain on the medial aspect of eyes and cheek. Stimulation of ostium (b) causes pain to be referred to the infraorbital and temporal regions (adapted from Wolff 1963).[145]

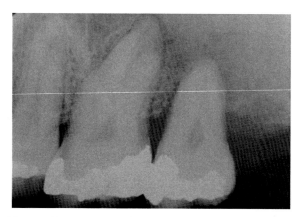

Fig. 16-4 Patient presented in acute pain of two weeks' duration. The maxillary second and third molars were vital, mobile and very tender to percussion. The patient was in severe pain. A diagnosis of acute maxillary sinusitis was made based on radiographic diagnosis.

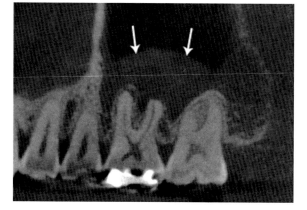

Fig. 16-5 Cone beam computed tomography (CBCT) images of lesion of endodontic origin from the non-vital maxillary first molar resulting in sinus mucositis, which is seen as a non-corticated thickening (arrows) of the sinus mucosa.

a unilateral maxillary sinusitis will have an odontogenic origin.[148]

Iatrogenic events such as extrusion of endodontic filling material, root fragments and other foreign bodies, and failure of a sinus lift procedure can damage the sinus lining and cause maxillary sinusitis.[149] Direct spread of pulpal and periradicular infections into the maxillary sinus is possible. The extrusion of endodontic filling material into the sinus may result in fungal infection that produces unilateral recalcitrant sinusitis.[150] Odontogenic cysts and tumors of the maxilla can also produce obstructive sinus symptoms.

Three varieties of odontogenic chronic sinus reactions are described:

1. Sinus mucositis
2. Odontogenic chronic maxillary sinusitis.
3. Fulminant acute odontogenic sinusitis.

Sinus mucositis

Sinus musocitis is defined as a reactive hyperplasia of the sinus mucosa of more than 4 mm thickness seen radiographically in proximity to an apical periodontitis associated with a maxillary molar or premolar (Fig. 16-5).[151] Sinus mucositis rarely produces symptoms of sinusitis. Roots of the offending teeth need not protrude into the sinus to produce these pathologic changes, as the porous cancellous bone provides an easy conduit into the sinus.

A periosteal reaction with new bone formation can occur around the mucosal thickening.[152] Periapical pathosis can also cause an elevation of the corticated floor of the sinus, which reduces the sinus volume and produces an *antral halo effect* on the sinus floor. This may be accompanied by symptoms of pulpal and periradicular disease, including toothache and pain on biting (Figs 16-6 to 16-8).[153] This condition can be radiographically distinguished from a mucous retention cyst, which does not have a radiopaque cortical outline. This differentiation is important as mucous retention cysts only occur within the mucosal lining of the sinus, are asymptomatic and do not require treatment.[153]

Odontogenic chronic maxillary sinusitis

Odontogenic chronic maxillary sinusitis (Figs 16-9 and 16-10) accounts for 10 to 12% of all cases of *chronic* maxillary sinusitis.[154] Patients present with symptoms that may include unilateral nasal discharge with foul odor or obstruction, changes in pain intensity with changes in atmospheric pressure, and a unilateral increase in maxillary pain on a sudden vertical change of posture.[147,153]

Odontogenic chronic maxillary sinusitis is frequently misdiagnosed and under-reported by radiologists.[155,156] A possible explanation for this is that "toothache" occurs in less than a third of these cases, whereas sinonasal symptoms are very common.[147] Thus, a thorough dental examination and careful

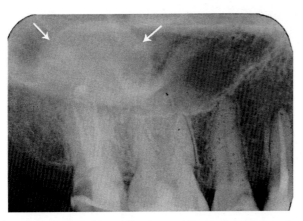

Fig. 16-6 An antral halo effect (arrows) due to the presence of a periapical lesion of endodontic origin on the maxillary right second molar showing a characteristic radiopaque outline.

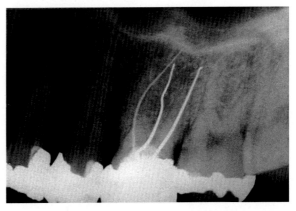

Fig. 16-7 Periapical radiograph of a patient who had persistent rhinosinusitis for 12 years, which resolved after the separated K-file was removed from the mesiobuccal canal during endodontic retreatment.

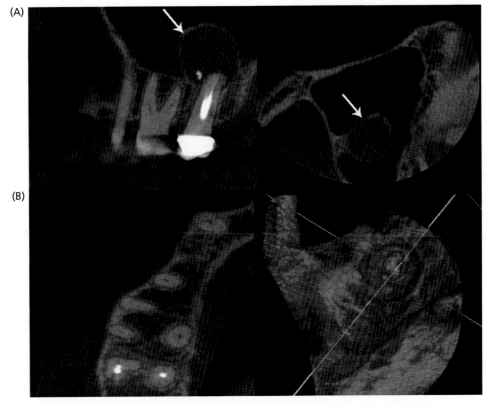

Fig. 16-8 CBCT images of the patient in figure 16-6. (A). The circumferential lesion of endodontic origin (arrows) expanding into the maxillary sinus can be seen. Note the corticated border around the halo and that the maxillary sinus is otherwise clear. The association of the lesion with the maxillary second molar can be seen. (B) Close examination of sagittal slices revealed a two-rooted molar with under-filled mesiobuccal root canals.

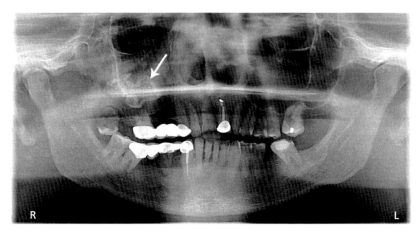

Fig. 16-9 A panoramic radiograph (OPG) showing radio-opaque foreign (endodontic filling material from a previously treated tooth that was extracted) material in the right maxillary sinus with sinus opacity (arrow). The maxillary sinus on the left is clear, while the one on the right is completely obstructed by the filling material and the mucositis associated with it. The maxillary right first molar was non-vital and may have contributed to the ongoing problems (see below).

(A)   (B)

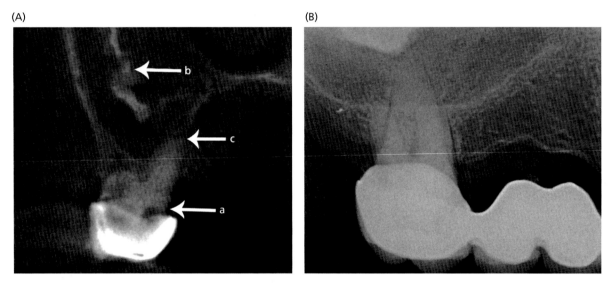

Fig. 16-10 Sagittal CBCT section (A) through the palatal root of the maxillary right first molar in Fig. 16-8A, showing a break in continuity of the palatal cortex at the root apex (arrow c) and the communication with maxillary sinus. Caries is seen as a radiolucency under the palatal margin of the crown (arrow a). The extruded filling material from extracted, previously endodontically treated teeth (arrow b) is clearly visible. Note the limited information provided by periapical radiograph (B) of the caries and the break in the continuity of the lamina dura.

reading of computed tomography (CT) scans are necessary before excluding odontogenic maxillary sinusitis as a diagnosis.[155] Studies show that periapical radiography detects one-third fewer periapical lesions than a CBCT examination, and that invasion of a lesion of endodontic origin into the maxillary sinus is difficult to diagnose by periapical radiography alone.[157]

Fulminant acute odontogenic sinusitis

Fulminant acute odontogenic sinusitis refers to maxillary sinusitis of odontogenic origin that spreads into other sinuses or intra-cranially.[158] More than one half of odontogenic maxillary sinusitis infections also involve the anterior ethmoidal sinus. Although rare, intracranial spread can occur. Symptoms such as altered mental state, headache and fever associated with a sinus infection should immediately alert the

clinician of the need for emergency treatment or expedited referral.[158]

Maxillary sinus disease may not be inflammatory. Space-filling lesions (e.g. maxillary sinus carcinomas) can cause obstruction of and pain in the sinuses (Fig. 16-11). These pathologic processes may mimic dental pathosis (Fig. 16-12).

Confirmatory tests for maxillary sinusitis

A careful clinical and radiological examination must be carried out to exclude a dental cause for maxillary sinusitis. The most important diagnostic test is pulp sensibility testing. Although radiographic and CT imaging may be helpful in confirming signs of rhinosinusitis, there is a lack of correlation between clinical symptoms, and endoscopic or CT scan findings.[159] Thus, the diagnosis is

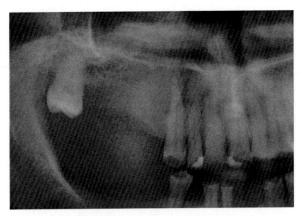

Fig. 16-11 A space-filling maxillary sinus carcinoma which presented for diagnosis as orofacial pain.

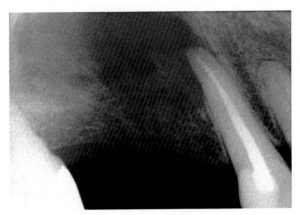

Fig. 16-12 Maxillary sinus carcinoma. The clinical and radiographic appearance mimicked an endodontic lesion. The irregular outline of the lesion and lack of healing after endodontic treatment should arouse suspicion of a non-dental cause.

often made from clinical observation and confirmed by the history and response to medication, especially decongestants.

Acute maxillary sinusitis is relatively easy to diagnose from its many signs and symptoms. The pain is often bilateral. Pain caused or increased by postural changes, infra-orbital palpation tenderness, and an unexplained sensitivity in maxillary teeth are all helpful diagnostic signs. A history of allergy, recent cold or fullness in the maxilla are also important indicators. If a maxillary dental examination, including pulp sensitivity testing, is negative for a dental cause of maxillary pain, particularly where several maxillary teeth are tender to percussion, practitioners should consider maxillary sinusitis, even when the classic signs and symptoms are absent.

Chronic sinusitis can be difficult to diagnose, although patients who present with chronic sinusitis are normally aware of their problem and are often under treatment. A close examination of the dentition is necessary in patients with unilateral chronic sinusitis. A CBCT examination is recommended if odontogenic chronic maxillary sinusitis is suspected.

A CT scan or an MRI is required if the patient does not respond to treatment with decongestants and antibiotics. These imaging tools are also indicated if a sinusitis complication such as osteomyelitis or abscess, or a condition that mimics sinusitis (e.g. neoplasm), is suspected.

When reviewing images, it is important to remember that a pathosis is evident only at the time the image was obtained. Imaging performed a few days after the signs or symptoms of a sinus infection have resolved may show little or no evidence of the original condition. Therefore, previous imaging is seldom useful for investigating a current sinus-related episode.

Treatment considerations

Dental treatment is indicated *only* if a dental problem is confirmed. An acute *toothache* or percussion sensitivity by themselves are *insufficient evidence* for dental intervention without further investigation.

The vast majority of acute rhinosinusitis infections are of viral origin, are self-limiting and resolve within 10 days. Decongestants and steam inhalation provide symptomatic relief in most patients. Topical decongestants generally should not be used for more than five days.[160] Nasal irrigation with saline is a safe alternative.[161]

It is important not to prescribe antibiotics for acute sinusitis unless:

- symptoms worsen after five days;
- there is a persistence of symptoms after ten days; or
- a bacterial origin is confirmed or suspected.[162]

Antibiotics and immediate referral are indicated in cases with orbital extension of sinusitis to prevent intracranial complications.

The widespread indiscriminate use of antibiotics is hypothesized as the reason for the development of antibiotic-resistant strains of bacteria. These resistant strains may be responsible for persistent sinus infection and development of chronic sinusitis.[163]

Chronic rhinosinusitis is considered an inflammatory disease of multifactorial etiology. Hence, treatment is focused on antimicrobial agents targeting the infection and other agents which modulate the inflammation.[160] Endoscopic sinus surgery may be needed for overall patient management. The microbiology of chronic rhinosinusitis is different from that of acute rhinosinusitis. Culture-directed antimicrobial therapy for weeks may be necessary for chronic rhinosinusitis.[160] The outcome of treatment is influenced by a patient's general medical and immune status, control of air quality and, when applicable, cessation of smoking.[160] Because chronic rhinosinusitis requires thorough medical assessment, an in-depth discussion of this condition and its treatment is outside the scope of this manual.

Treatment considerations for odontogenic maxillary sinusitis

Sinus mucositis of endodontic origin usually resolves with root canal treatment or extraction of the offending tooth. Resolution may take more than six months.[151] The initial treatment of severe *odontogenic* maxillary sinusitis, with obstruction of the ostium and complete obliteration of maxillary sinus with soft tissue, consists of removal of the dental cause by extraction of the offending tooth or elimination of the infection by root canal treatment. Broad-spectrum antibiotic therapy may be required for up to 3 months.[149] Referral to an oral and maxillofacial or ear, nose and throat (ENT) surgeon may be required for some odontogenic sinus infections. Significantly, the microbiology of odontogenic sinusitis is different from other forms of chronic sinusitis. It is polymicrobial and 50% anaerobic bacteria.[154]

Helpful questions to ask if you suspect a patient has pain from maxillary sinusitis

Does the severity of the pain change when you change your head position?

Postural changes influence the severity of pain. For example, lying on one side or the other, or bending down at the waist with the head tilted forwards.

Do you have a feeling of stuffiness or fullness in your face?

Sinus congestion will produce the stuffy or full feeling.

Do you get pain on both sides of your face?

Dental pain does not cross the midline. It is common for patients to have unilateral rhinosinusitis. Therefore, unilateral chronic maxillary sinusitis is often of dental origin.

Have you had cold or allergy symptoms lately, such as a cough or nasal congestion?

Upper respiratory symptoms may progress to sinusitis. *Hay fever* or acute allergic rhinitis may predispose to sinusitis.

Do your top teeth feel unusual?

Patients with maxillary sinusitis may report that their upper teeth feel *woody* or unusual, *similar to being anesthetized.* Firm bi-digital palpation of the alveolar bone above the apices of the maxillary molar teeth may elicit tenderness.

Are any of your teeth sore to biting or tapping?

Consider maxillary sinusitis when more than one *vital* maxillary tooth is sensitive to percussion.

Do you have headaches?

Patients can have pansinusitis (inflammation of *all* paranasal sinuses on one side or both sides). These patients complain of pain above the eyebrows or between the eyebrows and the bridge of the nose.

Do you have any tenderness in your face? Does it hurt when you press under your eye?

The overlying tissues of the face may be tender, particularly over the infra-orbital foramen.

Does your nose drip or have you noticed fluid dripping down your throat?

Post-nasal drip is a common symptom of sinusitis.

Do you get any relief of pain from a hot shower or decongestants?

Patients can get sudden, temporary pain relief if the ostium is unblocked.

Have you had a fever?

Fifty percent of adults and 60% of children have an elevated body temperature.

Have you been swimming lately?

Sinus congestion from swimming can precipitate maxillary sinusitis.

Have you had any problems with your sinuses before?

Chronic sinusitis waxes and wanes.

Has your sense of smell changed recently?

Patients with sinusitis often have a reduced olfactory sense.

Do you have any chronic illnesses?

Immunosuppressed or immunodeficient individuals are susceptible to chronic rhinosinusitis.

Chapter 17

Diagnosing Tension Headaches and Migraine

David Mock

Introduction

Headache is one of the most common symptoms or complaints.[164] While the most common causes of these are migraine and tension headache, there are many other causes (Table 17-1).[165] Chronic headache can arise from, but is not limited to, tension-type headaches, vascular disorders, neuralgias, intracranial infections (e.g. meningitis and encephalitis), space-occupying intracranial lesions (e.g. tumors), systemic diseases (e.g. thyroid disease and hypertension), giant cell arteritis, medication or substance withdrawal, post-traumatic headaches (head or neck injuries), cluster headache as well as migraine headaches. In some patients, vasoconstriction caused by *excessive smoking or caffeine intake* may be followed by a rebound dilatation, causing a *dull headache* (this is often relieved by further smoking or caffeine ingestion). Prolonged or intense exercise (especially in the presence of some additional factors such as high altitude) can result in the headache, which is similar to a migraine but does not last as long.

Clinically, many patients often report that they have *migraines*, but on questioning it becomes apparent that they are generalizing chronic headache with a diagnosis of migraine, a mistake often made by clinicians.

Most of these headaches are treatable and it is incumbent upon a practitioner to identify the type of headache described, and to refer the patient for appropriate treatment. Some headaches require urgent referral. It is therefore important to recognize headaches that do not fit the norm and that need referral for diagnosis and treatment, particularly, for example, if visual disturbances, systemic symptoms and jaw claudication are present.

Immediate referral is mandatory for patients who report first-time severe headache of increasing severity, as the possibility of an intracranial lesion has to be considered, particularly if other headache *red flags* are noticed.[166] These include systemic symptoms such as altered sensation or muscle dysfunction, headaches which are sudden onset (particularly in patients over 50), and/or where the headache is associated with nausea and vomiting, visual disturbance and/or pupillary asymmetry, seizures or collapse. It is not within the scope of this manual to discuss the management and treatment of these many different headache types. *Tension headaches and migraines are, however, discussed in detail.*

Tension-type headache[167–169]

Tension-type headache is the *most common headache* in adults and adolescents, while rare in children. There are many synonyms used for this type of headache, including *muscle contraction-type headache*. The headache is almost always *bilateral*. This helps to differentiate tension headache from cervicogenic pain which is usually unilateral. It is characterized by recurrent episodes of head pain with a pressing or tightening quality, sometimes described as the sensation of a tight headband or "vice-like." Headaches can last from half an hour to seven days or more. The pain is muscle based; however, muscle spasm has not been demonstrable as characteristic (myofascial TMD without limitation is similar).

The pathophysiology of tension headache is unknown; however, a peripheral trigger or multiple triggers are thought to initiate the process, and/or central sensitization. The onset can be triggered by stress, alcohol use, eye strain or fatigue. Unlike migraine headaches, *nausea and visual disturbances (aura) are not characteristic*, but can accompany the headache in severe cases. Light and noise can aggravate the headache. Tension-type headache can, and often does, *co-exist with myofascial TMD*.[170] The headache is not usually aggravated by normal movement.

Diagnosing Dental and Orofacial Pain: A Clinical Manual, First Edition. Edited by Alex J. Moule and M. Lamar Hicks.
© 2017 John Wiley & Sons, Ltd. Published 2017 by John Wiley & Sons, Ltd.
Companion website: www.wiley.com/go/moule/dental_and_orofacial_pain

Table 17-1 Simplified classification of types of headaches (modified from *The International Classification of Headache Disorders*, International Headache Society, 2013).[165,171]

Part I: The Primary Headaches
1. Migraine headaches
2. Tension type headaches
3. Cluster headache and other
4. Autonomic trigeminal cephalgias
5. Other primary headaches

Part II: The Secondary Headaches
6. Headache attributed to head and/or neck trauma
7. Headache attributed to cranial or cervical vascular disorder
8. Headache attributed to non-vascular intracranial disorder
9. Headache attributed to substance withdrawal
10. Headache attributed to infection
11. Headache attributed to disorder of homeostasis
12. Headache or facial pain attributed to disorder of cranium, neck, eyes, ears, nose, sinuses, teeth, mouth, or other facial and cranial structures
13. Headache attributed to psychiatric disorder

Part III: Cranial Neuralgias, Central and Primary Facial Pain and Other Headaches
14. Cranial neuralgias and central causes of pain
15. Other headache, cranial neuralgia, central or primary facial pain

---

Patients who experience tension headaches may get a premonition that one is about to occur, by a tightness in the shoulders or a soreness in the neck. A distinguishing feature between migraines and tension headaches is that migraines usually last for only a number of hours and they are often preceded by auras or visual disturbances, whereas tension headache can last for days. Nausea and vomiting are also a common feature of migraine. Migraines can precipitate a tension headache.[167,168]

Useful question to ask if tension headache is suspected

Can you show me with your hands where your head hurts?

Tension headache is usually bilateral, most often involving the temples, frontal and occipital regions, possibly extending into the back of the neck and shoulders. Patients usually use two hands to describe a tension headache pain and often circle the head or run their hands back and forth across the top of their head (see Chapter 6).

Where do you feel the pain starts?

The headache usually starts in the whole head or the back of the neck (occipital region).

What does it feel like?

Tightness or pressure sensations suggests tension-type headache.

Is there anything that brings on your headache?

Stress, anxiety, exertion or alcohol suggest tension-type headache. Also, poor posture and prolonged concentrated work can initiate the headaches.

Is there anything that relieves it or makes it less severe?

Relief from the application of heat (e.g. a hot shower or hot bath) or massage of the neck or scalp suggests tension-type headache.

How long does the headache last?

Tension headaches can last for days. This is a distinguishing feature that separates them from migraines.

Do you notice any other signs or symptoms such as visual changes, nausea or vomiting?

If nausea, vomiting or visual changes are reported, the patient is not suffering exclusively from a tension headache.

Confirmatory tests

- The history is suggestive of tension headache.
- There are usually tender points in the muscles of the scalp, face or neck.
- The pain does not usually disturb sleep.
- The neurological examination is negative.
- The pain generally responds readily to treatment.

NOTE: Patients with persistent tension-type headache should be referred for neurological examination. Imaging, particularly magnetic resonance imaging (MRI), is recommended to exclude intracranial-related abnormalities.

Treatment considerations[169,171]

Over-the-counter medication is preferred for short-duration and symptomatic relief (e.g. ASA, acetaminophen or ibuprofen):

- Physiotherapy and massage can be helpful if there are associated facial or neck symptoms.
- If a TMD is comorbid, collaboration between dentist and physician is recommended.
- Referral to a physician, ideally a neurologist, is recommended if the pain cannot be controlled.
- Cognitive behavioral therapy, mindfulness, relaxation and biofeedback can be helpful when pain cannot be controlled.
- A pain diary is useful to identify triggers and then to avoid them.
- In severe or resistant cases, and with medical consultation, tricyclic anti-depressants and selective serotonin reuptake inhibitors (SSRIs) can be prescribed.
- Botulin toxin injections have been suggested in severe unresponsive cases, but is an *off-label* (unapproved) treatment.

Migraine headache[167,168,172]

Migraine headaches tend to first occur between the ages of 10 and 45 and can run in families. The headaches can be triggered by stress, anxiety, strong odors, missed meals, noises, bright or flashing lights, physical activity, alcohol, some foods, sleep deprivation, caffeine withdrawal and, in women, changes in hormone levels associated with either menstruation or birth control pills. Some women notice a decrease in the incidence and severity of migraine headaches during pregnancy.

Typically, migraine headaches are often debilitating and start with a dull ache and then get progressively worse. *Visual disturbances* can precede the onset of the pain, including blurred vision, seeing stars and flashes, tunnel vision or a temporary blind spot. The headaches have a *pounding, throbbing or pulsating nature*, and they are *unilateral* and behind the eye, or *bilateral* but worse on one side of the head. Headaches rarely last more than 48 hours, with *most lasting for a number of hours* only. Patients often report *sensitivity to light and sound*. Symptoms can be *aggravated by movement*.

Migraine can be classified as with or without aura. It can co-exist with temporomandibular pain that, in turn, could be a risk factor for increased headache frequency and for the development of chronic migraine. Allodynia (pain due to a stimulus that does not normally provoke pain) is more prominent when the two conditions co-exist.

Migraine is further subdivided into chronic migraine and episodic migraine, a distinction important in deciding on an appropriate management plan. Generally patients who have up to 14 headache days per month are considered to have episodic migraine versus those with more than 14 headaches per month, who are classified as having chronic migraine.

There are a variety of theories regarding the pathophysiology of migraine headaches as well as subclassifications. It is generally recognized that migraine headaches are caused by abnormal brain activity, but the precise pathophysiology is unclear.[173] An intracranial vascular basis is widely accepted but, more recently, it has been demonstrated that the pain is centered in the trigeminal complex of the brain stem.

Useful questions to ask if migraine headache is suspected

Where do the headaches occur?

Migraines tend to be worse on one side of the head with pain behind the eye or in the back of the head.

How do the headaches start?

Migraines usually start as a dull ache and with visual disturbance if with aura.

Describe the headache?

Migraines exhibit a throbbing, pounding or pulsating sensation.

How long does a headache last?

These generally last for 6 to 48 hours.

Is there anything that initiates your headaches?

There is often a trigger, but they also can appear to start spontaneously.

Do you have any other symptoms, apart from the pain?

Migraines are generally accompanied by one or more of the following: sensitivity to light or noise, nausea or vomiting, chills, fatigue, loss of appetite, altered sensation or sweating.

Confirmatory tests and clinical findings

- The diagnosis is primarily based on the history.
- Physical examination should be carried out to eliminate other local causes such as infection, eye disorders, sinus or dental disease.
- If a TMD is comorbid, collaboration between dentist and physician is ideal.[173] Referral to a physician, ideally a neurologist, is recommended.
- Brain imaging, generally MRI, is often carried out to rule out a space-occupying lesion.
- Electroencephalography (ECG) should be taken to rule out seizure disorder.

Treatment considerations

- Medication for an acute attack includes triptans, analgesics and non-steroidal anti-inflammatory drugs (NSAIDs).
- Administration of riboflavin (vitamin B_2) (400 mg/day) has been shown to reduce the frequency and severity of migraine attacks.[174]
- Referral to a physician, preferably a neurologist, is recommended.
- Behavioral approaches such as cognitive-behavioral therapy (CBT) and Mindfulness are useful for preventive management.
- Preventive medications include tricyclic amines, antihypertensive, anticonvulsants and botulinum toxin injections.
- If the migraine is comorbid with TMD, addition of physiotherapy, rest, heat (carefully applied), stabilizing appliance if indicated and muscle relaxants can be helpful.
- Botulinum toxin injections are used for refractory cases.

Chapter 18

Diagnosing Cluster Headaches

Kerryn Green

Introduction

Cluster headaches are the most frequent type of headaches belonging to the group known as the trigeminal-autonomic cephalalgias. These are primary, *unilateral* headaches that occur with cranial autonomic symptoms.[175] They are characterized by *excruciating pain in the region of the trigeminal nerve* (usually orbital or peri-orbital). While the pain is almost exclusively unilateral during the attack, it may shift sides within a cluster (see video 18.1).

Cluster headaches occur predominantly around the eye and the temporal region but may radiate to the jaws and teeth (upper > lower).[176] These severely painful headaches recur in clusters lasting weeks to months. Each separate attack builds up to a peak usually within 10 to 15 minutes and lasts 15 minutes to 3 hours. Within the cluster most patients have one or two attacks daily. The pain usually occurs around the same time each day and often will wake the patient from sleep. Remissions of a few months to years may occur.

The pain is usually described as excruciating, with a boring, piercing, stabbing, tearing or burning character. Often the sufferer will pace the floor and sit up in a posture that provides maximal relief. Cluster headache is most often abrupt in both onset and ending.

Associated autonomic symptoms

The typical cluster headache is associated with cranial autonomic features, which almost always occur *unilaterally* on the same side as the pain (Fig. 18-1). These features may include:

- Conjunctival injection (significant vasodilation of conjunctival blood vessels causing the eye to appear red)
- Lacrimation (excessive tearing of the eye)

- Rhinorrhea (nasal discharge) or nasal congestion
- Horner's syndrome: unilateral ptosis and miosis (drooping of the eyelid and constricted or small pupil) (Fig. 18-2).

Prevalence

Although cluster headache is relatively rare in the general population, some epidemiological studies show the prevalence may be as high as one person per 500.[177] It is more common in men than in women (4:1).[178] Although it can begin at any age, most patients report symptoms starting in their 20s or 30s.

Cause

Cluster headache is a primary headache disorder, which means there is no known structural cause. The pathophysiology of cluster headache is not clearly understood.

Triggers of acute cluster attacks include alcohol (usually within an hour of intake, but not in periods of remission), elevated environmental temperature, exercise and nitroglycerine medications.

Diagnosis

The diagnosis is made after a careful history and examination are obtained and other structural causes are excluded. The history is easily recognizable. The following criteria (Table 18-1) have been established in the International Classification of Headache Disorders for a diagnosis of cluster headache.[179]

Because cluster headache is frequently misdiagnosed, the condition is incorrectly treated. Indeed, studies have shown that it may be many years before patients are diagnosed.[180] As dentists may be the first professional contact for these patients, it is important

Diagnosing Dental and Orofacial Pain: A Clinical Manual, First Edition. Edited by Alex J. Moule and M. Lamar Hicks.
© 2017 John Wiley & Sons, Ltd. Published 2017 by John Wiley & Sons, Ltd.
Companion website: www.wiley.com/go/moule/dental_and_orofacial_pain

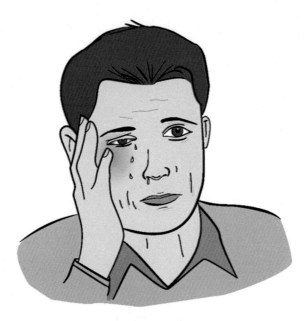

Fig. 18-1 A patient with cluster headache. Note the unilateral nature of the pain, Horner's syndrome, redness of the eye, redness on the cheek and nasal discharge.

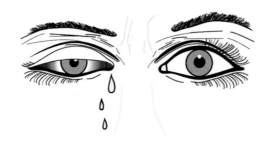

Fig. 18-2 Diagrammatic representation of a patient with cluster headache exhibiting Horner's syndrome. Note the unilateral drooping (ptosis) of the eyelid and constricted pupil (miosis) as well as the tearing and the sub-conjunctival injection (red eye).

Table 18-1 Criteria necessary for a diagnosis of cluster headache (adapted from International Classification of Headache Disorders).[165]

A. At least five attacks fulfilling criteria B–D
B. Severe or very severe unilateral orbital, supraorbital and/or temporal pain lasting 15–180 minutes (when untreated)
C. Either or both of the following:
  1. At least one of the following symptoms or signs, unilateral to the headache:
    a) conjunctival injection and/or lacrimation
    b) nasal congestion and or rhinorrhea
    c) eyelid oedema
    d) forehead and facial sweating
    e) forehead and facial flushing
    f) sensation of fullness in the ear
    g) miosis and/or ptosis
  2. Sense of restlessness or agitation
D. Attacks have a frequency between every other day or up to 8 per day for more than half the time when the disorder is active.
E. Not better accounted for by another diagnosis.

to be aware of this condition and refer the patient to their general medical practitioner.

Similar to many other *intermittent pains,* diagnosis of cluster headache is difficult as it may not be present when the patient appears for a consultation. It is helpful to ask the patient to return during a cluster headache attack or even to provide a photograph on a mobile phone of themselves during an attack so that any associated signs, including redness of the eye and Horner's syndrome, can be seen and recorded. The associated nasal congestion can be confusing and can result in a mistaken diagnosis of sinusitis or allergies.

Other serious conditions may present with similar features to cluster headache and need to be excluded. These include an inflammatory or neoplastic process involving the cavernous sinus or pituitary fossa. An MRI brain scan, sometimes together with a computed tomography (CT) scan of the base of skull, is required to diagnose these conditions. Vascular pathologies such as aneurysm, arterio-venous (AV) malformation or carotid dissection (see Chapter 21) can be ruled out with MRI angiography. Horner's syndrome is also a feature of carotid dissection (a tear in the wall of the artery), which may occur spontaneously or as a result of neck trauma or manipulation. This causes a false lumen to form which may fill with clotted blood. Subsequently, a blood clot may dislodge and cause a stroke. Thus, if signs and symptoms, which include sudden onset of prolonged head and neck pain, visual or speech disturbances or limb weakness or tingling, suggest a carotid dissection, immediate referral to a neurologist is indicated.[181]

Other primary headaches (headaches without a structural cause) that may present similar symptoms to cluster headache include other trigeminal–autonomic cephalalgias. Paroxysmal hemicrania is an important condition to recognize, as it responds promptly to indomethacin, which is not the case in other trigeminal-autonomic cephalalgias. Paroxysmal hemicrania attacks usually occur with high frequency (mean frequency is 14 attacks per day)[182] and are shorter in duration than those of cluster headaches. They lack the circadian periodicity of cluster headaches, and alcohol is an infrequent trigger.[183] It is important that practitioners look at the patterns that these painful conditions present. When these patterns are not recognized, preventing the development of a sound treatment plan, then the patient should be referred to a specialist for consultation and treatment.

Useful questions to ask if cluster headache is suspected

Where is the pain?
Cluster headache always occurs on one side of the face, usually in and around the eye.
How would you describe the pain?
Patients usually describe the pain as hot, searing, pricking or drilling, rather than dull or aching.

How often do you get the pain?

The pain occurs from once every other day to three attacks per day. The clusters of attacks may last weeks to months with remission lasting months to years.

How long does the pain last?

Each headache period lasts 30 minutes to 2 hours.

At what time of the day do most of your headaches occur?

Most cluster headaches occur at night, waking the patient from sleep. This is unlike trigeminal neuralgia or migraine, which commonly occurs during daylight hours. Generally, neuralgias do not wake people at night.

How severe is the pain?

Cluster headache pain can be excruciating.

Do you feel like going to bed with the pain?

Patients having a cluster attack are often restless and agitated and will pace around the room. Unlike migraine headache, the pain is not exacerbated by movement.

Do your eyes water or become red when you have the pain?

Patients with cluster headache often develop excessive lacrimation (tearing) and conjunctival redness.

Is the pain accompanied by nasal stuffiness or nasal drip?

Patients often report nasal congestion with cluster headache.

Does your top eyelid droop on the same side of the face as the headache?

Patients often develop unilateral ptosis with cluster headache.

Does light bother you when you have the headache?

Photophobia may occur with the headache; however, other migraine-associated features such as nausea, vomiting or the migraine aura are absent.

Are you able to get relief from the headache with pain pills such as Panadol (acetaminophen) or aspirin?

These non-narcotic analgesics are usually ineffective in relieving cluster headache pain.

Does alcohol make the pain worse during your headaches?

Alcohol exacerbates the headaches during a cluster period, but rarely precipitates an attack during a period of remission.

Have you had any recent neck trauma or pain, weakness, or changes in sensation in your arms or legs?

Carotid artery dissection can mimic the pain and ptosis of cluster headaches. Carotid dissection must be excluded if there are symptoms of neck pain or muscle weakness, altered sensation in the extremities or a history of neck injury or manipulation.

Confirmatory tests

A typical history and appearance of a patient suffering from cluster headache should confirm the diagnosis. Blood tests and radiological imaging are not useful in diagnosing cluster headache. MRI/ MRA or CT scans may be necessary, however, to rule out other pathology such as carotid artery dissection or other structural lesions.

Treatment considerations

Acute treatment

- Oxygen 100% administered through a facial mask at a rate of 7 L/min for 15 min is often effective at relieving the headache.
- Triptan medications (e.g. Sumitriptan 6 mg subcutaneously), which are used for acute treatment of migraine, are usually effective.
- Prednisone may be used to suppress the cluster. It is usually started with 60–80 mg per day and tapered off over 2 weeks.

Preventative treatment

- Verapamil, a calcium channel blocker used in the treatment of hypertension, is commenced at diagnosis and increased as needed.
- Lithium, which is used in the treatment of bipolar psychiatric disease, may be effective.
- Topiramate, an anticonvulsant used in the treatment of epilepsy, may be effective. It is started at low doses and increased as needed.

Chapter 19

Diagnosing Trigeminal Neuralgia

Kerryn Green

Trigeminal neuralgia

Trigeminal neuralgia (TN) is a neuropathic pain condition involving the trigeminal nerve (Cranial Nerve V). It is caused by an injury to or a lesion of the nerve. It is characterized by recurring bouts of excruciating pain in the face. The pain is described by patients as brief, sharp, electric shock-like, jabbing, stabbing, searing or burning. The pain lasts for a few seconds to several minutes. Multiple attacks can occur in a short period of time. In between the severe paroxysms of pain, there may be a lingering ache in the facial region. The bouts of pain are often separated by long periods of remission.

TN occurs in one or more of the three branches (V1, V2, V3) of the trigeminal nerve (Fig. 19-1). The characteristic feature of this pain condition is the presence of trigger points, which can be activated by light touch or movement. Typical examples of these triggers include brushing the teeth, shaving, talking, eating, or having cold water or cold air contact the face. Infrequently trigger points can be on the teeth. Pain is often accompanied by an involuntary movement of the face, described historically as a tic. TN is almost always unilateral.

The incidence of new cases of TN in the general population is 12/100 000 per year. TN is more common in patients older than 50, with 60 years of age reported as the average. As patients age, the bouts of pain may become more frequent and severe.[184]

Cause

The most common cause of TN is thought to be compression of the trigeminal nerve root close to its entry into the pons.[185] In the majority of cases, an aberrant artery, usually the superior cerebellar artery, compresses the trigeminal nerve at the pons as it arises from the brainstem.[185,186] As patients age, blood vessels elongate and the brain *sags* causing aberrant blood vessels.[186] The pulsatile vascular compression by these aberrant blood vessels causes an abnormal generation of sensory impulses.

Diagnosis

In most patients TN is fairly easy to diagnose based on a typical history. Special attention, however, should be given to patients who have symptoms that include permanent facial numbness or weakness, have an atypical presentation such as bilateral TN or are younger than 50 years. This heightened caution is indicated because these atypical types of TN can be a symptom of an underlying major pathology.

Other causes

Other causes of TN that are very serious or life-threatening include an aneurysm or arteriovenous (AV) malformation, tumors or an inflammatory lesion associated with multiple sclerosis.[187] The prevalence of TN in multiple sclerosis patients is 20 times greater than in the general population.[188] Multiple sclerosis is the most common neurological condition affecting young adults.

Pre-trigeminal neuralgia

Sometimes patients experience a prodromal orofacial pain in the teeth or jaws, termed *pre-trigeminal neuralgia*, which may last minutes to hours. It can be triggered by jaw movements or drinking hot or cold liquids. It has been shown to eventually convert to typical TN within days or even years later.[189] Of particular importance is that in its early stage pre-trigeminal neuralgia can mimic toothache. Even experienced practitioners can make mistakes in the diagnosis of these patients. All too frequently, patients with

Diagnosing Dental and Orofacial Pain: A Clinical Manual, First Edition. Edited by Alex J. Moule and M. Lamar Hicks.
© 2017 John Wiley & Sons, Ltd. Published 2017 by John Wiley & Sons, Ltd.
Companion website: www.wiley.com/go/moule/dental_and_orofacial_pain

(A)   (B)

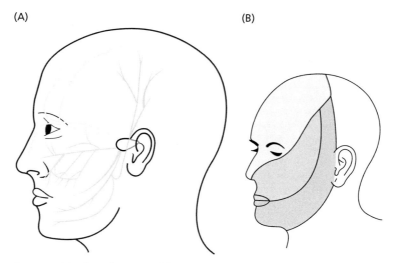

Fig. 19-1 Distribution and course of the three divisions of the trigeminal nerve. The ophthalmic branch (V1) (blue) conducts sensation from the scalp, forehead, front of nose and eye. The maxillary branch (V2) (lavender) conducts sensation from the cheek, upper jaw, top lip, gingiva and alveolar mucosa, maxillary teeth and the side of nose. The mandibular branch (V3) (ocher) conducts sensation from the lower jaw, mandibular teeth, lower lip, gingiva and alveolar mucosa.

pre-trigeminal neuralgia are subjected to multiple dental procedures in a well-intended but unsuccessful attempt to relieve the pain.[190] Early recognition of this pain, with the appropriate referral and medications, can avoid unnecessary and often irreversible procedures.

NOTE: Be aware of dental-type pain that does not add up, particularly if the descriptors used by the patient are uncharacteristic of dental pain, for example jangling, burning, jolting or electric shock-like.

The symptoms of pre-trigeminal neuralgia are not usually the sharp, electric shock-like pain characteristic of classic TN. Patients often remember the exact day when their pre-trigeminal neuralgia converted to trigeminal neuralgia.

Glossopharyngeal neuralgia

Although TN is uncommon in the general population, it is the most common neurological condition encountered by most dentists.[190] A similar but very rare condition, glossopharyngeal neuralgia (pain due to pathology of Cranial Nerve IX), exhibits the same unilateral sharp, electric shock-like, jabbing, stabbing or burning pain that lasts for seconds to minutes. The pain can radiate to or from the posterior tongue, pharynx, ear or lower jaw. Its triggers are swallowing, chewing, talking, coughing or yawning. The pain also may be triggered by sweet, cold, hot or acidic food or liquids. Sometimes just touching the ear or side of the neck can trigger the pain. Pain can be relieved temporarily by a topical anesthetic spray applied to the throat. Although the most common cause of glossopharyngeal neuralgia is an aberrant blood vessel compressing the nerve, other lesions, particularly those that involve the brainstem, need to be excluded.

Useful questions to ask if trigeminal neuralgia is suspected

What sort of pain are you having?

Brief electric shock-like or stabbing pain is strongly suggestive of TN.

How often do you get the pain?

Pain from TN is characterized by many short, sharp jabs of pain.

How long does the pain last?

Pain from TN rarely lasts more than 30 seconds to a minute.

Does anything set off or trigger the pain?

Touching the face, exposing the face to wind or cold water, shaving, chewing and talking are triggers for TN.

Where is the pain?

TN always occurs along one or more divisions of the trigeminal nerve (Fig. 19-1).

On a scale of 1 to 10, where 10 is the most severe pain you can imagine, how severe is your pain?

TN patients invariably rate their pain as 9 or 10 out of 10.

Does the pain wake you up?

The pain usually does not wake the patient at night.

Is the pain present when you wake up, or does it occur after you wake up?

Patients usually wake up pain free, but experience pain once they start to talk or eat.

Is the pain constant or do you have pain-free periods?

TN occurs as bouts of intense pain usually followed by pain-free periods. When asked, patients may recall a similar problem occurring in the past.

Have you had a similar pain in the past?

Multiple episodes of TN may occur with some frequency. Conversely, the patient may have long periods of remission in between episodes.

Do mild analgesics such as paracetamol (acetaminophen) or non-steroidal anti-inflammatory agents (aspirin or ibuprofen) relieve the pain?

Non-opioid analgesics rarely relieve the severe pain of TN.

Is your pain on just one side or on both sides of your face?

Bilateral pain is very uncommon in TN. When it does occur it is usually found in another family member with a familial trait for TN or from a secondary cause such as a pontine lesion in the brainstem (e.g. multiple sclerosis).

Is the pain getting more intense with each episode or is it the same each time?

Worsening symptoms increase the possibility of a structural lesion (e.g. a tumor) causing the pain.

Have you noticed any other signs or symptoms such as difficulties in swallowing, facial weakness or changes in vision or hearing?

TN can be a symptom of an underlying disease such as multiple sclerosis, a space-occupying lesion or an abnormal anatomical structure compressing or infiltrating the nerve.

Confirmation tests for trigeminal neuralgia (TN)

Because the diagnosis is almost always made clinically rather than by laboratory tests or imaging, a typical history is the most important confirmation of TN. Therefore, blood tests or radiological imaging are not required to confirm the diagnosis. When tests or imaging are used, they serve to exclude other causes, particularly when there are atypical features in the history or examination.

A patient with typical TN may be hypersensitive on the surface of the face on the same side as the pain. Atypical features include lack of sensation, reduced movement of the face or other abnormal cranial nerve signs:

- Magnetic resonance imaging (MRI) may be performed to exclude a compressive or inflammatory brainstem lesion (Fig. 19-2) or other inflammatory lesion (e.g. multiple sclerosis) (Fig. 19-3).

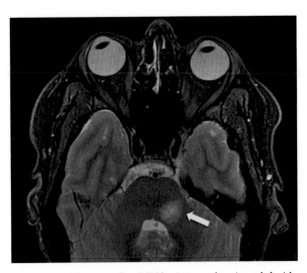

Fig. 19-2 Axial image of an MRI brain scan showing a left-side lesion (arrow) in the pons within the brainstem.

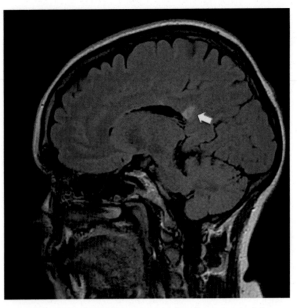

Fig. 19-3 Sagittal MRI brain image showing a typical deep cerebral white matter lesion (arrow) seen in a multiple sclerosis patient. TN is often associated with multiple sclerosis.

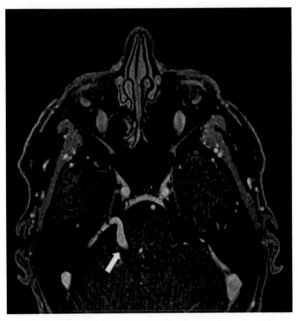

Fig. 19-4 Axial MRI showing the anterior superior cerebellar artery compressing the trigeminal nerve close to where the nerve arises from the pons in the brainstem.

- Magnetic resonance angiography may show a blood vessel (usually the anterior superior cerebellar artery) compressing the trigeminal nerve close to the nerve root entry zone at the pons in the brainstem (Fig. 19-4).
- The pain of TN is typically relieved by neuropathic pain medications (e.g. carbamazepine or gabapentin).
- A referral for a neurological consultation is usually required to confirm the diagnosis and for subsequent patient management.

Treatment options

Medication is the first-line therapy for TN because of its proven success in treating the pain. Medications commonly used are Tegretol® (carbamazepine), Lyrica® (pregablin), Neurontin® (gabapentin) and Lamictal® (lamotrigine).

In some patients, medications are ineffective or not tolerated due to side effects.[191] There are surgical options for these cases:

- A *destructive* procedure where the sensory function of the trigeminal nerve is intentionally eliminated (via freezing, gamma knife radiosurgery, alcohol or glycerol injections).
- A *non-destructive* procedure where the nerve is decompressed and its sensory function is usually preserved (microvascular decompression). The surgical procedure is tailored to the patient and their risk profile.

Microvascular decompression is the most popular surgical treatment due to more favorable long-term results and the lower risk of sensory loss in the face.[192,193] This procedure involves surgery via an incision behind the ear to locate and mobilize the aberrant blood vessel that is compressing the trigeminal nerve as it arises from the brain stem. A Teflon® sponge is placed between the vessel and the nerve to maintain separation of the two structures, which decompresses the nerve (Fig. 19-5).

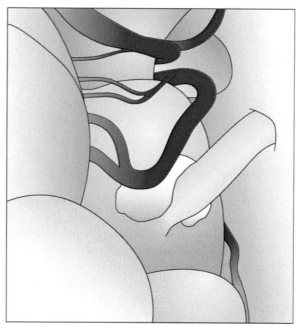

Fig. 19-5 Microvascular decompression surgery in which a Teflon® pad (blue) has been placed between the trigeminal nerve (TN) and an aberrant artery (red) close to where the nerve arises from the brainstem (adapted from: https: http:// neurosurgery.ufl.edu/patient-care/diseases-conditions/ trigeminal-neuralgia/Accessed 29 July 2015).

Chapter 20

Viruses as a Cause of Orofacial Pain

Michael J. Apicella

Viral infection as an etiologic source of orofacial pain

The most common of these infections are caused by the herpes simplex viruses 1 (HSV1) and 2 (HSV2). HSV1 is more commonly associated with oral infections[194] and is the primary infection usually seen in children and young adults. Oral infections result in blisters or balloon-like vesicles accompanied by fever, malaise, regional lymphadenopathy and difficulty in eating (dysphagia). Symptoms usually resolve in two weeks. The virus then moves to a sensory nerve ganglion where it remains as a latent or dormant virus. Reactivation of the virus results in a herpes simplex labialis infection (cold sore), which responds in its early stages to antiviral creams.[195] All herpes virus infections are highly contagious and spread by direct bodily contact with an infected person or through airborne respiratory secretions.

Varicella zoster virus

Of the eight known herpesviruses that infect humans, *varicella zoster virus (VZV)* may be diagnostically the most challenging. The virus is a common childhood virus that is responsible for the cutaneous vesicular skin eruptions commonly known as *chicken pox*. The infection causes fever and malaise, and manifests as a vesicular skin rash with itching on the face and body for several days. This is followed by scabbing of the vesicles and eventual resolution of the signs and symptoms after one to two weeks. As the condition resolves, the virus becomes dormant in the dorsal root ganglia and is contained by the body's cell-mediated immunity. Later in life, reactivation of the VZV can occur with the appearance of painful blisters known as herpes zoster, zoster or "shingles."

Orofacial herpes zoster (shingles)

VZV emerges in a unilateral distribution in one of the primary sensory nerves from the reactivation of dormant virus particles in a dorsal root or cranial nerve ganglion.[196] This may occur due to a decrease in the patient's cell-mediated immune system because of increasing age, medications, malignancy, stress or trauma. VZV infections result in a dermatomal distribution of blistering skin eruptions. Although any sensory ganglion and its cutaneous nerve can be involved, lesions most commonly form on the thoracic, lumbar and cervical regions of the body (Fig. 20-1).[197]

Of special interest is that VZV can manifest in the trigeminal nerve (CN V) up to 15% of the time, resulting in orofacial pain. Although any one of the three divisions of CN V can be involved, usually it is only one, with the most common being the ophthalmic division (Fig. 20-2).[198]

The emergence of VZV usually manifests itself in several stages.[199] Initially, there is usually a distinctive prodromal pain that will be felt in the affected dermatome. It is in the first stage or prodromal phase that the patient first notices the symptoms of herpes zoster (HZ). In the area of the face, this is along the distribution of one of the three divisions of the trigeminal nerve (CN V) or the facial nerve (CN VII). It can occur several days before the appearance of the vesicles and can be severe. It has been described as itching, burning, tingling, boring, prickly or knife-like. There can also be headache, allodynia or a non-painful altered sensation.

NOTE: Pain from HZ may initially occur as a new-onset toothache. Before the vesicles erupt, this toothache may last a few days or be delayed for up to 7 months.[200–202]

The next stage is considered the "acute phase." The characteristic dermatomic rash appears on the

Diagnosing Dental and Orofacial Pain: A Clinical Manual, First Edition. Edited by Alex J. Moule and M. Lamar Hicks.
© 2017 John Wiley & Sons, Ltd. Published 2017 by John Wiley & Sons, Ltd.
Companion website: www.wiley.com/go/moule/dental_and_orofacial_pain

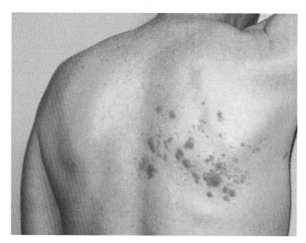

Fig. 20-1 Photograph of a patient suffering from VZV infection two days after the first vesicles were noticed. The patient suffered severe local pain, altered sensation and allodynia along the distribution of the thoracic nerve trunk.

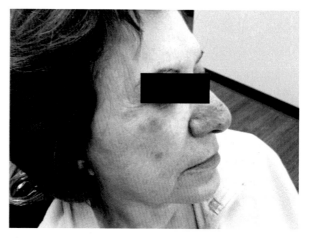

Fig. 20-3 Patient with HZ (V2) of CN V who presented with severe headache above the eye and in the temple area prior to vesicles appearing. Vesicles then appeared several days later. **Note**: Vesicles are confined to the distribution of the maxillary division (photograph courtesy of Dr Curt Warren).

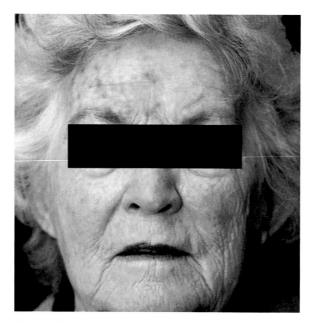

Fig. 20-2 Patient with severe headache above the right eye and in the temple area prior to vesicles appearing. A diagnosis of HZ was made when vesicles appeared several days later. **Note**: Vesicles are confined unilaterally to the distribution of the ophthalmic division (V1) of the nerve.

skin or in the oral cavity, and the pain severity increases. The patient may also complain of malaise, headache, nausea and low-grade fever. The initial rash or papules can become vesicles within 12 to 24 hours (Fig. 20-3), followed by pustules in 1 to 7 days. As well as being painful, they can become unbearably itchy. Severe allodynia is common.

At 7 to 8 days the pustules begin to dry out and crust. The crust will normally fall off within 14 to 21 days.[199] Occasionally scar tissue may form once the scabs have resolved, and is characterized by hyper- or hypo-pigmented skin lesions. The pain from HZ usually resolves once the lesions heal. In approximately 10% of cases, the pain will persist and the condition enters a chronic painful phase. This is referred to as post-herpetic neuralgia (PHN). There can also

be dental complications, which have been reported to result from a facial herpes zoster. These include tooth devitalization (multiple teeth developing necrotic pulps),[203] tooth exfoliation, internal root resorption, odontalgia, and osteonecrosis of the mandible.[204] Permanent eye damage or even blindness can occur if vesicles form on the surface of the eye.[198]

Although HZ typically goes through a phase in which vesicles occur after the prodromal phase, in rare instances the patient may develop pain without the eruption of vesicles. This is known as *zoster sine herpete*.[205] Complications of VZV infection can include Guillain-Barré syndrome, encephalitis, myelitis, Ramsay Hunt syndrome, and ocular complications including ulcerations, hemorrhage, conjunctivitis and optic neuritis.[205]

Diagnosing facial herpes zoster

Facial HZ can be readily diagnosed once the vesicles are seen with their characteristic dermatomal distribution. In the prodromal stage, it is necessary to first rule out pain of odontogenic origin by assessing the vitality and radiographic integrity of each tooth on the affected side. An absence of temperature sensitivity in the presence of severe pain mimicking toothache suggests a non-dental cause. The pain descriptors used by the patient to describe the typically unilateral pain are *atypical for dental pain*. Descriptors likely to be used by the patient include *itching, burning, sharp, stabbing* or *throbbing*. In addition, normally innocuous stimuli produce pain (allodynia).

Where no obvious dental or other cause can be established, no treatment except for pain control with analgesic medications should be carried out. The patient should be placed under close observation. Once the vesicles do appear, the diagnosis should be straightforward. The patient should be referred immediately for antiviral medication.

Useful questions to ask the patient for facial herpes zoster (shingles) of CN V

What sort of pain have you been having for the past few days?

Although HZ of the trigeminal nerve may appear as a toothache in the prodromal stage, be cautious in your diagnosis if the descriptors used (e.g. itching, burning, sharp or stabbing) are not characteristic of dental pain.

Are you experiencing any sensitivity to heat or cold?

It is unusual to have severe and prolonged dental pain without the commonly associated signs and symptoms, including temperature sensitivity.

Is the pain constant or does it vary?

A characteristic of pulpal pain is that it varies over time and is not constant.

Where are you experiencing the pain?

Pain from HZ (shingles) will follow the distribution of one of the three divisions of the trigeminal nerve. The pain and dermal distribution of VZV infection should also differentiate HZ from the ulcerations caused by the herpes simplex virus (HSV).

Have you ever had chicken pox?

HZ results from a reactivation of VZV from the primary episode of chicken pox

Are you feeling tired, have a fever, or experiencing headaches?

Reactivation of the virus can occur when host defences are compromised. Patients with HZ will often show some systemic symptoms including tiredness, headache and fever. In the absence of overt signs of a dental infection, a non-dental cause should be suspected.

Do you have any medical conditions that may affect your immune system?

Are you taking any medications that may affect your immune system?

Have you recently experienced an increase in stress?

Reactivation of the virus can occur during times of stress because of its suppressive effect on the immune system.

Confirmatory tests for herpes zoster

The diagnosis of HZ is usually made easily once vesicles appear. Laboratory tests are only indicated where a herpes simplex virus (HSV) infection should be ruled out or for atypical lesions (e.g. for immunocompromised patients where the course of the disease is prolonged or unusual,[206] or if *zoster sine herpete* is suspected). Laboratory testing using DNA from the patient's blood along with polymerase chain reaction (PCR) or direct immunofluorescence assay can aid in the diagnosis of VZV infection.[197] The effectiveness of laboratory testing to identify HZ in the prodromal phase of the infection has not been established.

Treatment considerations for herpes zoster

Although HZ is a self-limiting disease, complications such as PHN can be reduced with the use of antiviral medications such as acyclovir (e.g. Zovirax®),

valacyclovir (Valtrex®) and famciclovir (Famvir®). However, in order to get maximum benefit from these medications, they need to be administered within 72 hours of the onset of the rash.[197] Vaccination with Zostavax® against shingles for patients age 50 or older has been shown to prevent (~50% effectiveness) or reduce the incidence and severity of the infection.[207]

Currently there are no interventions that can effectively treat or control the pain of HZ.[209] Analgesics such as paracetamol (acetaminophen) or ibuprofen in combination with codeine may help. Frequently, stronger analgesics may be needed. Emollient and anti-inflammatory creams and ice packs can be effective in reducing the severe pain and allodynia. Patients with facial VZV infections involving the eye should be referred *immediately* for medical evaluation and treatment, as permanent damage can occur if the surface of the eye is involved.

Patients with facial HZ can become completely debilitated, as eating and drinking may be very difficult for them. Care must be taken to ensure that a patient maintains an adequate fluid intake and does not become dehydrated.[208]

Ramsay Hunt syndrome

Ramsay Hunt syndrome consists of the triad of facial paralysis, ear pain, and herpetic eruptions in any cranial dermatome.[209] The syndrome occurs when the virus reactivates from latency in the geniculate ganglion and affects cranial nerve VII and associated cranial motor nerves following the distribution of the nervus intermedius.[210] The symptoms of Ramsay Hunt syndrome are very similar to those of Bell's palsy, except for the occurrence of vesicles that commonly occur in and around the ear and the mouth.[211] In addition, these patients may suffer from vertigo, hearing loss, tinnitus, severe otalgia and the inability to close the eye on the ipsilateral side.[209] Severe pain may be the first symptom to occur, followed by vesicle formation and finally facial paralysis. Significant oral findings include lesions on the anterior two-thirds of the tongue and the soft palate.[210] Infrequently, Ramsay Hunt syndrome may also occur without the eruption of the vesicles and is known as *zoster sine herpete*. In this case, Bell's palsy will need to be part of the differential diagnosis. Without the vesicular eruptions, serological or molecular methods may be needed to make the final diagnosis.[209] The prognosis for complete recovery from the facial paralysis of Ramsay Hunt syndrome is not as good as for Bell's palsy.[211]

Useful questions to ask if Ramsay Hunt syndrome is suspected

NOTE: Refer first to questions above for trigeminal nerve HZ.

Have you had pain in the side of your face?

Ramsay Hunt syndrome can be accompanied by severe debilitating pain along the distribution of the facial nerve (CN VII).

Have you noticed any blisters appearing on the side of your face?

In Ramsay Hunt syndrome vesicles follow the distribution of the facial nerve, which innervates the whole of the side of the face and ear.

Do you have pain or ringing in your ear?

The facial nerve innervates the stapedius muscle of the middle ear. Tinnitus is a common symptom of Ramsay Hunt syndrome.

Are you experiencing any problems with balance?

Patients with Ramsay Hunt syndrome also report problems with their equilibrium or balance.

Do you have pain in the front half of your tongue?

The facial nerve conducts taste sensations from the anterior two-thirds of the tongue.

Do you have any facial weakness?

The facial nerve controls the muscles of facial expression.

Post-herpetic neuralgia

PHN follows HZ in approximately 10% of all cases.[196] However, the incidence increases with age and can affect up to 73% of the elderly.[196,212,213] A diagnosis of PHN may be made when the pain persists from HZ for three months or longer. Risk factors include advanced age, severe prodromal pain, severe HZ pain and rash.[213,214]

The pain in PHN is unilateral and occurs in the region of the vesicular eruptions, although the distribution can be wider. It can be described as itching, burning, sharp, stabbing or throbbing. Allodynia *and* hyperalgesia may be present, or conversely, decreased sensitivity and numbness have been reported. The pain may be either spontaneous or stimulus dependent. The likelihood of developing PHN is significantly higher with HZ infections in the trigeminal dermatomes[196] and in the ophthalmic region than in other areas.[214] In the elderly population, depression is a concern with individuals who experience debilitating and long-term pain.[199] Unfortunately, the pain of PHN can last a lifetime. Proper management, however, can reduce pain and suffering and ultimately improve the quality of life in these patients.

Useful questions to ask if PHN is suspected

Have you suffered from shingles?

Almost all patients with facial shingles will remember the event.

Have you suffered painful blisters in the last several months on the side of your face?

PHN occurs within the same dermatome or sensory nerve involved with the VZV infection. The discreet scarring that occurs after resolution of the HZ rash may aid in the diagnosis of PHN.

Have you ever had the shingles vaccine?

Vaccination with Zostavax against shingles for patients 50 years or older reduces the risk of PHN after shingles by over 60%.

Confirmatory tests for orofacial PHN

Confirmation is obtained via a history of continuous pain in an area previously affected by shingles, often with associated allodynia or hyperalgesia.

Treatment considerations for orofacial PHN

In addition to the protracted pain of PHN, the condition often leads to depression, disrupted sleep and decreased functioning. Therefore, treatment of PHN is problematic as the complication often does not respond to normal analgesic strategies. Complementary combinations of medications are usually required, including gabapentin and tricyclic antidepressants and pregabalin, topical lidocaine patches and opioids. An in-depth discussion of treatment of PHN is beyond the scope of this manual. Readers are referred to current guidelines on the care of PHN.[215]

Chapter 21

Vascular Causes of Headaches

Mark Paine

Giant cell arteritis

Giant cell arteritis (GCA), otherwise known as temporal arteritis or cranial arteritis, is a medium- to large-sized vessel vasculitis occurring in patients over the age of 50 years. It is the commonest vasculitis in this age group. The incidence increases with increasing age, with most patients being over the age of 60 years. GCA can occur in any of the cranial arteries. It is important to consider this in a differential diagnosis of any patient presenting with unexplained orofacial or craniofacial pain, because it can be associated with significant but preventable morbidity including blindness and stroke.[215,217] With appropriate and timely treatment, GCA is treatable and often curable. Some of the symptoms of GGA are given here.

Headache

Headache and facial pain are present in most, but not all, patients. Although the headache can be severe and disrupt sleep at night, it can also be relatively mild and non-specific. Sometimes neck pain is more prominent than headache.

Systemic symptoms

Tiredness, night sweats, fever, weight loss or loss of appetite can be a feature. Most patients have at least one sign or systemic symptom.

Tenderness

There may be focal pain or tenderness over the scalp in the region of the superficial temporal arteries. There may also be associated nodular swelling or enlargement of the superficial temporal arteries, often accompanied by a reduced or absent pulse (Fig. 21-1). The scalp or temporal tenderness may result in difficulty in washing or brushing the hair. On occasion, patients may have difficulty putting their head on a pillow, wearing a hat or brushing their hair because of the extreme temporal tenderness.

Visual disturbances

Loss of vision is a feared complication of GCA. Patients may report episodes of transient vision loss before a permanent loss of vision. If the diagnosis is made following a transient episode, permanent vision loss may be averted with appropriate and timely treatment. The estimates of frequency of vision loss vary; however, 15 to 20% of patients develop profound vision loss in one or both eyes. This occurs as a result of occlusive disease involving the posterior ciliary circulation or the central retinal or ophthalmic arteries (Figs 21-2 A and B). Once loss of vision occurs in one eye, it is permanent, and vision loss in the other eye usually ensues within days or weeks.

NOTE: Any patient who presents with orofacial pain and also reports visual disturbances must be *immediately* referred to a neurologist or an ophthalmologist to exclude the possibility of GCA causing sudden blindness.

Claudication

Pain or aching in the muscles of mastication can occur in up to one-third of patients.[218] Claudication refers to pain and cramping in muscles that gradually develop during exercise, but eases when the muscles are

Diagnosing Dental and Orofacial Pain: A Clinical Manual, First Edition. Edited by Alex J. Moule and M. Lamar Hicks.
© 2017 John Wiley & Sons, Ltd. Published 2017 by John Wiley & Sons, Ltd.
Companion website: www.wiley.com/go/moule/dental_and_orofacial_pain

rested. Jaw claudication is a sign of GCA, occurring in up to half of sufferers. This symptom is the result of inflammatory stenosis of the branches of the maxillary artery. The pain may not be localized to the jaw muscles, but also can involve the tongue or throat. It can be mistaken for temporomandibular joint (TMJ) dysfunction.[219]

NOTE: Unexplained TMJ pain in an older patient should raise the suspicion of GCA.

Localized ischemic complications

Although not common, localized ischemic complications can result if GCA is not recognized early. Ischemic complications, such as scalp or orolingual ulceration or necrosis, may also occur less frequently (Fig. 21-3).[220–223] Transient or persistent *diplopia* can result from ischemia to cranial nerves or the extra-ocular muscles. Up to 20% of patients can have occult GCA, a variation of the condition where an ischemic complication, usually vision loss, occurs.

Involvement of the extra-cranial vertebral arteries may result in occipital ischemia/infarction in the absence of a systemic disturbance (Fig. 21-4).[224–226]

In summary, GCA should be suspected if there is a new onset of orofacial, cranial or cervical pain in a patient over the age of 50 years, especially if:

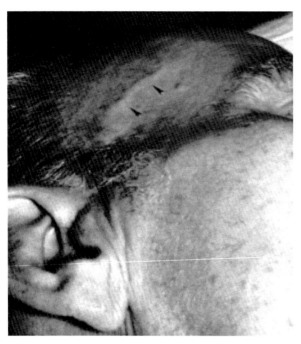

Fig. 21-1 Tender and prominent temporal artery (arrows) in a 65-year-old man who experienced sudden loss of vision in his right eye. Blood tests revealed an elevated erythrocyte sedimentation rate (ESR) and biopsy showed evidence of GCA (reproduced by permission from *Walsh and Hoyt's Clinical Neuro-ophthalmology* (2006), Lippincott: Williams & Wilkins).

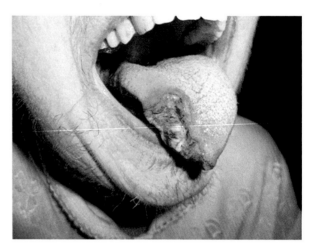

Fig. 21-3 Ischemic complication involving lingual ischemia and infarction (from N. Mumoli, M. Cei, J. Vitale, F. Dentali (2015) *Tongue Necrosis in Giant-cell Arteritis*. DOI: 10.1093/qjmed/hcv099. First published online: 15 May 2015).

(A)

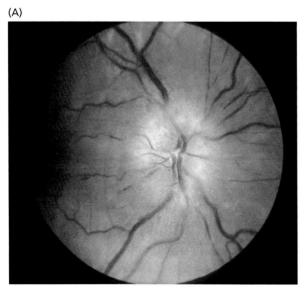

(B)

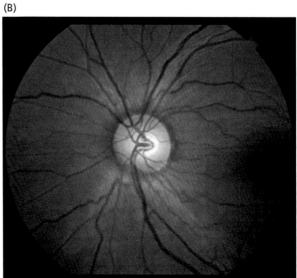

Fig. 21-2 Retinal photograph depicting normal eye (A) and the swollen optic disc associated with anterior ischemic optic neuropathy (B) (courtesy Dr Neil Shuey).

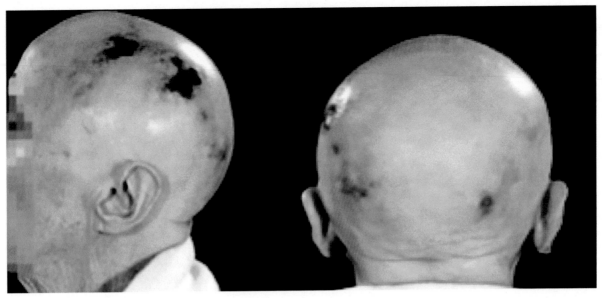

Fig. 21-4 Ischemic complication involving the extra-cranial vertebral arteries resulting in occipital ischemia and infarction (reproduced from Morris *et al.* 2006 *Clin Experi Ophthalmol* with permission).

- symptoms are suggestive of jaw, oral or lingual claudication.
- systemic symptoms are present (e.g. fever, sweats, anorexia, appetite loss, weight loss or polymyalgia).
- there is a history of a previous (and often recent) otherwise unexplained transient or permanent loss of vision or diplopia.

NOTE: GCA responds dramatically to prednisone. If there is a strong suspicion of GCA, especially in patients with visual changes, the immediate administration of prednisone, 1 mg/kg body weight per day, is indicated to prevent irreversible blindness secondary to occlusion in the ophthalmic circulation.

Questions to ask if giant cell arteritis is suspected

Have you been feeling sick recently?
Have you noticed any fever or night sweats?
Have you noticed any loss of appetite or loss of weight?

Systemic or constitutional symptoms may be prominent in some patients with GCA. On careful questioning, the majority of patients will admit to having at least one systemic sign or symptom.
Have you recently developed a headache or facial pain?
Have you experienced any unusual neck pain?

Headache and neck pain are common symptoms in GCA. However, there are no specific features of headache and neck pain that suggest the diagnosis. It is the clinical context of the signs and symptom(s) that is important, including the age of the patient (most are over 60 years) and elevated Erythrocyte sedimentation rate (ESR) levels.
Have you had any pain or tenderness over your temples?

Tenderness over the temporal area raises the suspicion of GCA in certain contexts, but is not specific to the condition.

Have you noticed any difficulty with your vision recently, such as double vision, blurring or loss of vision in one or both eyes?

Pay strict attention to any patient who presents with both *orofacial pain and visual disturbances*. The occurrence of transient or permanent loss of vision or diplopia in these patients *strongly indicates a medical emergency*. Visual symptoms confer a high risk of permanent loss of vision in the unaffected eye in the short term if urgent treatment is not provided. While treatment may not salvage vision that has already been lost, timely treatment may prevent further deterioration of vision or the occurrence of other ischemic complications.
Have you had any cramping or aching in your jaw or mouth when you chew?

Jaw claudication or related oro-mandibulo-lingual variants are suggestive of GCA and are associated with an increased risk of ischemic complications. Jaw claudication is a feature in up to one-third of patients with GCA. When claudication is suspected in patients who report pain on eating, care should be taken to first exclude TMD as a diagnosis. Conversely, care should be taken to include GCA in the differential diagnosis in elderly patients who present with symptoms suggestive of TMD.
Have you noticed any recent muscle or joint aches or pains, for example in the neck, shoulder or hip? Has there been any muscle or joint stiffness, particularly in the morning?

These symptoms are suggestive of a systemic disease such as *polymyalgia rheumatica*, which is found in approximately 50% of patients with GCA.
Have you noticed any ulcers or sores on your scalp?

Scalp ulceration fortunately occurs infrequently, but is dramatic and associated with an increased risk of ischemic complications and a poor prognosis.

(A) (B)

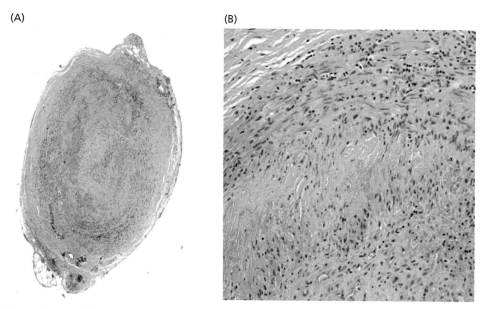

Fig. 21-5 (A) Photomicrograph of temporal artery showing transmural inflammation (original magnification 40×). (B) Obliteration of the arterial lumen by thrombosis and inflammatory tissue (original magnification 200×) (courtesy of Dr P. McKelvie, St Vincent's Hospital, Melbourne).

Confirmatory tests

The comprehensive assessment of patients suspected of GCA requires a synthesis of a multitude of discrete pieces of information, rather than relying on any single clinical feature or test result. The initial investigation is easy and non-invasive, involving a full blood examination (FBE). ESR and C-reactive protein (CRP) are the most commonly used inflammatory markers. Although they are not specific, the ESR and CRP are often markedly elevated in GCA. However, malignancy, infection or other inflammatory conditions also can cause these markers to be elevated.

There is no single confirmatory test, except for an abnormal temporal artery biopsy, which will show inflammation (Fig. 21-5). Infrequently, a bilateral biopsy is required.

While the need for temporal artery biopsy is sometimes questioned, most practitioners who deal with patients with ischemic complications of GCA would consider a temporal artery biopsy mandatory if the clinical picture is strongly suggestive for the condition. Frequently, however, the results of the biopsy may be inconclusive or even negative. Sometimes diagnostic confirmation can be difficult despite the above assessments. Further investigation using fundus fluoroscein angiography, positron emission tomographic (PET) scan or biopsy of another cranial artery (e.g. the occipital artery) may be required.[216] Other types of vasculitis can cause headache and facial pain. These include Kawasaki disease, Wegener's vasculitis, polyarteritis nodosa and vasculitis associated with other rheumatological disorders. They also include Takayasu disease, a similar disease to GCA with a very different demographic profile (e.g. a young Asian woman under

the age of 40 years). These are much less common causes of vascular cranio-facial pain, which are beyond the scope of this chapter.

Treatment considerations

Suspicion of GCA requires urgent treatment, even before investigation is completed. Steroids are often started before temporal artery biopsy. GCA responds dramatically to high-dose steroids which should be administered at the same time as the patient is having blood drawn for ESR and CRP. The steroid of choice is Prednisolone 1 mg/kg/d.

Any suspicion of vision involvement requires urgent ophthalmic or neuro-ophthalmic assessment for signs of ocular ischemia. Patients with established or threatened vision loss require IV steroids, which usually involves emergency hospital admission. This situation may arise during follow-up of the patient. It may indicate an inadequate level of immunosuppression or other treatment, or a flare-up of disease activity.

Cranial (carotid) artery dissection

Cranial artery dissection results from a rupture or tear of the intima layer of a cranial artery resulting in intra-arterial mural hematoma formation. Subsequent extension of the dissection can lead to occlusive thrombosis or embolism with associated complications from ischemic and/or compression of local neural structures. The condition can occur spontaneously or may result from trauma or existing arterial disease such as fibromuscular dysplasia.[227,228] The internal carotid artery is the most frequently involved artery.

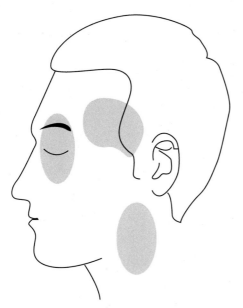

Fig. 21-6 Distribution of pain in patients suffering from a carotid dissection.

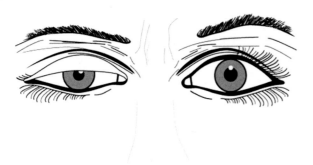

Fig. 21-7 Horner's syndrome, a sign of carotid dissection, involves ptosis (drooping of the lower eyelid) and miosis (constriction of the pupil) on the same side.

Patients with cranial artery (especially carotid) dissection may present with ipsilateral headache and orofacial or cervical pain, which are usually severe and of sudden onset. The pain often involves the neck, jaw, face, ear, peri-orbital or fronto-temporal regions (Fig. 21-6).

Signs and symptoms may also include transient monocular visual disturbance and unilateral Horner's syndrome (*ptosis*, drooping of the lower eyelid, and *miosis*, constriction of the pupil) (Fig. 21-7).

Horner's syndrome results from compression of the ascending cervical sympathetic nerves which course along the carotid artery.[229] Carotid artery dissection should be considered initially in any patient presenting with a painful Horner's syndrome. The pupillary miosis may be more evident in low ambient lighting conditions.

Embolization of the ophthalmic/retinal arteries may result in transient ipsilateral monocular vision loss or permanent vision loss caused by central branch retinal artery occlusion. *Ipsilateral* cerebral hemispheric embolization may result in transient or permanent cerebral ischemia with associated *contralateral* hemiparesis, facial paresis, hemisensory disturbance or dysphasia.

Cranial artery dissection is estimated to cause up to 25% of strokes in younger patients.[230] The compressive effects of carotid dissection may also cause lower cranial nerve palsies, most commonly hypoglossal palsy due to the proximity of these nerves to the carotid sheath, resulting in speech disturbances.[231]

A diagnosis of carotid dissection is difficult to make in the context of an isolated recent-onset headache/orofacial pain/cervical pain. It would normally be the occurrence of pain in association with the other clinical features which would lead to the suspicion of this clinical diagnosis. The outcome is variable. Most patients recover completely. Some remain with severe permanent deficits. Urgent referral to a neurologist is necessary if this condition is suspected.

Questions to ask if cranial nerve dissection is suspected

Have you noticed any headaches, facial pain or neck pain recently?

Although there is no specific pattern of pain, the majority of patients will present with acute-onset unilateral headache, facial pain or cervical pain.

Have you noticed that one of your eyelids is droopy?

Approximately 50% of patients will develop Horner's syndrome with mild unilateral ptosis and miosis.

Have you noticed any temporary or permanent loss of vision in one eye?

Have you noticed any temporary or persistent disturbance of your speech?

Have you noticed any temporary or persistent weakness or numbness of one side of your body or face?

Ischemic symptoms, which may present as unilateral loss of vision, disturbances in speech patterns or cerebral symptoms including facial numbness or paralysis, may develop within hours or even days after the onset of the dissection.

Have you noticed any difficulties with swallowing or with your tongue or voice?

The compressive effects of carotid dissection may cause lower cranial nerve palsies, most commonly hypoglossal palsy due to the proximity of these nerves to the carotid sheath. This leads to disturbances in tongue movements and speech patterns.

Confirmatory tests

Imaging is required to evaluate and confirm the clinical suspicion of carotid artery dissection. Ideally, these involve cranial and cervical magnetic resonance imaging or angiography (MRI/MRA). Because MRI/MRA images are more sensitive, they may also reveal the signature intramural arterial hematoma (a bright

(A)

(B)

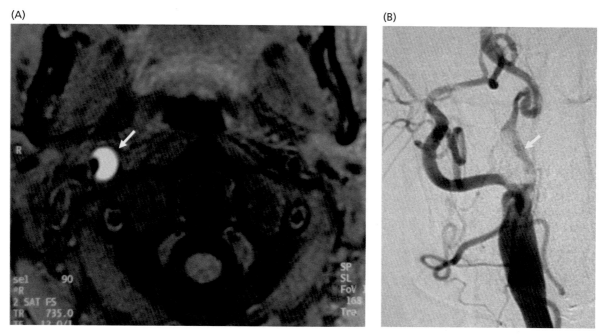

Fig. 21-8 MRI/MRA of brain (A) revealing the signature intramural arterial hematoma (arrow). A bright crescentic signal change within the carotid artery wall can be seen on this fat-suppressed T1-weighted image. (B) Digital subtraction angiography showing narrowing of the dissected carotid artery (images courtesy of Dr N. Trost).

crescentic signal change within the carotid artery wall on the fat-suppressed T1-weighted imaging) (Fig. 21-8). CT angiography or carotid Doppler ultrasonography can also show the characteristic morphology of carotid stenosis.

Treatment considerations

Immediate referral is indicated. Initial medical management may involve intravenous and oral administration of anticoagulants or antiplatelet agents.

Chapter 22

Diagnosing Neuropathic Orofacial Pain

E. Russell Vickers and Alex J. Moule

Types of neuropathic orofacial pain

Pain is a highly personal, unpleasant experience for a patient, yet it is invisible to the clinician. It is a highly conserved, basic survival instinct that informs higher centers of the brain to assess the situation and seek relief. Orofacial pain can be acute or chronic. Acute pain often occurs as a result of trauma, injury or a disease such as cancer or infection. However, in some circumstances acute pain may progress to persistent chronic pain, even after acute inflammation resolves with treatment. This type of pain, which accompanies neurogenic (nerve-induced) inflammation, can present confusing symptoms and can only be diagnosed with proper attention to the patient's history of pain. When diagnosing these unusual pain problems, physicians and dentists must obtain as much accurate and germane information as possible to render a correct diagnosis. Otherwise treatment will fail, especially when trying to distinguish dental pain from pain of non-dental origin (e.g. trigeminal neuropathic orofacial pain).

Neuropathic pain involves the expression of pain producing neuropeptides, including substance P and other neurokinins.[232] These neuropeptides are resistant to enzymatic breakdown, causing chronic neuropathic pain. This pathological process requires different treatment approaches, frequently involving anti-neuropathic drugs. It also presents in other parts of the body in the form of *phantom limb* (amputation) pain, *post-herpetic neuralgia* of the thorax, *failed back surgery syndrome* and *complex regional pain syndrome* (previously termed reflex sympathetic dystrophy).

Examples of neuropathic orofacial pain are:

- Burning mouth syndrome
- Trigeminal neuropathic orofacial pain
- Atypical odontalgia (also known as phantom tooth pain)[233,234]
- Post-herpetic facial neuralgia
- Atypical trigeminal neuralgia.

NOTES:

- Many patients are very familiar with the nature and cause of their pain and volunteer a large amount of information. Nevertheless, their descriptions of the pain may not be accurate. Be aware of patients who present a long history in a historical or diagnostic fashion, rather than giving you factual information.
- In the diagnosis of acute orofacial pain, listen carefully to *facts about the pain* rather than problems resulting from the pain, such as the inability to go to work.

The term atypical facial pain (AFP), which formerly was used to describe complex facial pains, is no longer in vogue. Its use implied, *"I do not know!"* (the cause of this pain). Unusual or atypical pain can result from many undiagnosed conditions, including pathology, neurological conditions, or muscle dysfunction. They can also result from a neuropathic orofacial pain or occasionally psychiatric disorders. Both the International Headache Society (IHS) and the International Association for the Study of Pain (IASP) have adopted the term "persistent idiopathic facial pain (PIFP)" to replace AFP. PIFP is defined as "persistent facial pain that does not have the characteristics of the cranial neuralgias [...] and is not attributed to another disorder."[235]

There are many trigeminal pain states to consider when developing a differential diagnosis of trigeminal neuropathic facial pain. They include:

- Dental pain caused by caries, pulpitis, abscess or cracked tooth (see Chapter 12)
- Pathology such as maxillary sinus disease or oropharyngeal cancer

Diagnosing Dental and Orofacial Pain: A Clinical Manual, First Edition. Edited by Alex J. Moule and M. Lamar Hicks.
© 2017 John Wiley & Sons, Ltd. Published 2017 by John Wiley & Sons, Ltd.
Companion website: www.wiley.com/go/moule/dental_and_orofacial_pain

- Oral mucosal pain from aphthous ulcers or oral lichen planus (see Chapter 3)
- Neurological disorders including headache syndromes (see Chapters 16, 18, 19 and 21)
- Myofascial pain (temporomandibular disorder) (see Chapter 14)
- Cervicogenic pain
- Cervical spine degeneration can cause mandibular pain. In addition to the mandibular division of the trigeminal nerve, the dorsal sensory roots of C2–C4 innervate the inferior border of the mandible (see Chapter 15).
- Cardiac pain referred to the mandible and chin (from myocardial infarction and coronary artery disease)
- Psychiatric conditions involving deliberate self-trauma.

Clinical presentation of neuropathic orofacial pain

Neuropathic orofacial pain is usually constant and moderate to severe in intensity. However, the presentation is varied:

- The condition varies frequently from low intensity in the morning to higher intensity in the evening, typically ranging from 5 to 8 on a scale of 10 (VAS). *Mild pain in the morning* results from the production of endorphins (pain-reducing endogenous opiod peptides) during sleep. *Increased pain in the evening* is caused by an increase in the level of pain-producing, neurotransmitters including substance P and epinephrine.
- The pain has *specific qualities* including burning (C-fiber activation) and sharp, shooting neuralgic pain (A-delta fiber). There also can be aching and throbbing qualities (Figs 22-1 a and b).
- *Local anesthetic* (LA) injections *do not work* or are only partially effective. LA agents such as lignocaine, prilocaine and mepivacaine block sodium channels to prevent nerve conduction. Neuropathic pain often involves the loss of the magnesium ion plug from the calcium channel; thus, pain persists despite numbness from the LA block.
- A clinical examination is normal and radiographs show no pathologic changes, but there is severe pain! Neuropathic pain occurs at the molecular level involving altered cell receptors and pain peptides. It cannot be directly observed by a practitioner or by the use of a mirror, probe or radiographs.
- *Dental stimulation*, including thermal and mechanical, rarely affects the pain.
- The patient can be *totally convinced* that the pain is coming from a tooth and can point out the exact tooth or area they consider to be responsible for the pain.
- Patients will *demand* that treatment be initiated or continued.
- Repeated dental treatment fails to resolve the pain.

- Most patients with atypical odontalgia will have multiple dental procedures completed before an accurate diagnosis is reached.
- The pain has been *present for months or even years* before diagnosis. It rarely resolves without treatment with anti-neuropathic medication.
- Neuropathic trigeminal orofacial pain usually has an initially narrow, well-defined pain field (*starts in one tooth*), but *then spreads* over a period of weeks or months to create a much wider pain field (*involves more teeth*).
- Conversely, acute dental pain may initially present in a wide field with pain that is *diffuse and difficult to localize*. It then shrinks to a single offending tooth that has caries, a crack or other causes like a symptomatic pulpitis.
- *Medications* such as paracetamol (acetaminophen), codeine, tramadol and even morphine *do not reduce the pain*. These medications are only effective on classical inflammation, not neurogenic inflammation. Medication for neuropathic pain typically requires amitriptyline (a tricyclic antidepressant), gabapentin or pregabalin (anticonvulsant), and topical capsaicin (common name: cayenne pepper), which depletes substance P.
- Eventually *pain can cross the midline* of the face due to central nervous system (CNS) *maladaptive neuroplasticity*. Clinically, the pain often spreads to multiple intra-oral sites involving teeth and mucosa (Figs 22-2 and 22-3).

There may be an associated *dysesthesia* (pain in an area of altered sensation), primary and *secondary hyperalgesia* (an increased response to a painful stimulus) and *allodynia* (pain to a stimulus that normally does not produce pain). For example, a primary state of neuropathic pain often causes *secondary myofascial pain* and *sympathetically maintained pain*. This is explained by the projections of the trigeminal nerve that extend to the brain stem and spinal cord with interneuronal connections to other nerve pathways (activation of motor nerves and the sympathetic nervous system) (Fig. 22-4).

The patient may present with *diagnostic pain states* in the oral and facial region, which include:

- *Sympathetic nervous system hyperfunction*, characterized by episodes of swelling and redness in the cheek or cheeks (termed sympathetically maintained pain) (Fig. 22-5) and *secondary temporomandibular disorder* with bilateral jaw/face pain (Fig. 22-6).
- Persistent pain causes *depression, anxiety and frustration*. Studies show up to 75% of patients with neuropathic pain of the trigeminal nerve have a moderate to severe psychiatric diagnosis, often due to the unremitting pain.[236]
- Dental treatment following an *episode of prolonged personal stress* or long-term worry or anxiety can be a factor in the initiation of neuropathic pain. Precipitating factors may include dental infection, endodontic therapy and maxillofacial trauma.

34. What makes your pain worse ? (fill in more than one circle if applicable)

- ● sitting
- ○ lying down
- ○ working
- ○ exercise
- ○ everything
- ○ household chores

- ○ rest
- ○ weather changes
- ○ hot weather
- ○ cold weather
- ○ heat applications
- ○ cold applications

- ○ pressure
- ● touch
- ● stress
- ● noise
- ● negative thoughts
- ○ social activities

35. What makes your pain better ? (fill in more than one circle if applicable)

- ○ sitting
- ● lying down
- ○ working
- ○ exercise
- ○ everything
- ○ household chores

- ○ rest
- ○ weather changes
- ○ hot weather
- ○ cold weather
- ○ heat applications
- ● cold applications

- ○ pressure
- ○ touch
- ○ distractions
- ○ being busy
- ○ positive thoughts
- ○ social activities

36. Please select from the list below words that you would use to describe your pain.* Fill in one circle for each word to indicate the intensity of each word where:

⓪ = not present   ① = mild   ② = moderate   ③ = severe

Quality of your pain	not present	mild	moderate	severe
throbbing	⓪	①	②	●
shooting	⓪	①	②	●
stabbing	⓪	①	②	●
sharp	⓪	①	②	●
cramping	⓪	●	②	③
gnawing	⓪	①	②	●
hot-burning	⓪	①	②	●
aching	⓪	①	②	●
heavy	⓪	①	②	●
tender	⓪	①	●	③
splitting	⓪	①	●	③
tiring-exhausting	⓪	①	②	●
sickening	●	①	②	③
fearful	⓪	①	●	③
punishing-cruel	⓪	①	②	●

Fig. 22-1 Pain qualities and location of the orofacial pain of a 68-year-old female with a 10-month history of pain after dental treatment in the right maxilla. Pain intensity was described as 8–9/10 (VAS). A diagnosis was made of primary neuropathic pain and secondary onset of temporomandibular disorder myofascial pain (from *Short-form McGill Pain Questionnaire* and excerpt from *Clinical Pain Inventory* in Vickers, R.D. Harris, H. Boocock and M.K. Nicholas (2006) *Orofacial Pain Problem Based Learning*. Sydney University Press 2005 Vickers (ed.), pp. 30–50).

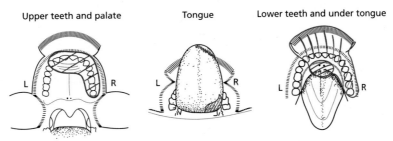

Fig. 22-2 Intra-oral pain map of the above patient. Pain was initially in the right mandible and then spread to the tongue and left orofacial region. Pain intensity 8/10 (VAS). A diagnosis of primary neuropathic pain was made. The expansion of the pain field to other teeth and across the midline illustrates CNS maladaptive neuroplasticity.

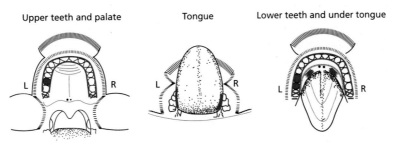

Fig. 22-3 Intraoral pain map of a patient diagnosed with trigeminal neuropathic orofacial pain demonstrating maladaptive neuroplasticity of all quadrants and bilateral borders of the tongue.

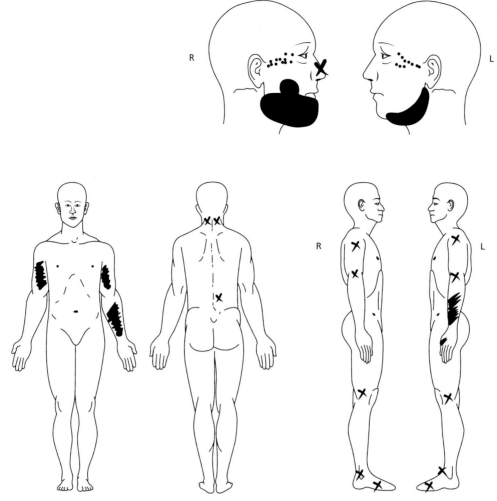

Fig. 22-4 Extra-oral pain map of patient illustrated in Figs 22-1 and 22-2 showing spread of pain to extra-oral sites in the extremities, neck and back. The patient was also previously diagnosed with fibromyalgia. The multiple pain sites as represented in this figure of both neuropathy and fibromyalgia have central sensitization phenomena.

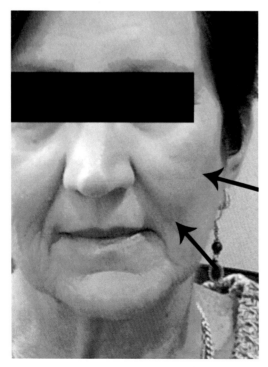

Fig. 22-5 Upregulation of the sympathetic nervous system. Note swelling and redness in the left cheek (arrows) in a patient with trigeminal neuropathic orofacial pain that developed after root canal treatment root canal therapy (RCT) of her maxillary left canine tooth.

Diagnosing the pain problem

The diagnosis of neuropathic pain is difficult as the symptom of pain is invisible. Diagnosis requires a careful, detailed approach. It is important that practitioners act as a diagnostician first to assess and then diagnose a condition *before* they become surgeons and provide treatment that may be irreversible. It is important to allow the patient to state the full scope of their pain problem.

It is important to remember that pain causes suffering and psychological distress. The physiological component of pain is only part of the "pain phenomenon." Because anxiety about not having a diagnosis also can increase the intensity of pain, providing a diagnosis alone can be beneficial in reducing pain. Reassuring the patient that they are in the care of a knowledgeable and empathetic practitioner reduces anxiety, which in turn can reduce the amplification of pain.

It is sometimes difficult to obtain meaningful information about pain from the patient. Thus, a pain consultation has to take the form of a carefully constructed interview to identify the physiological components (pain described as *burning or sharp*), the psychological components (pain described as *cruel or*

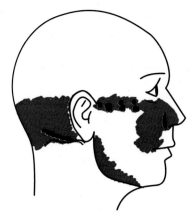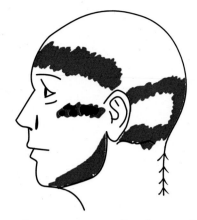

Fig. 22-6 Secondary development of bilateral myofascial pain involving the masseter, temporalis and supraspinal muscle groups. A patient has marked the right cheek (black) as the initial source of neuropathic pain following trauma to the right infra-orbital nerve. The other red areas are insertions of muscle groups.

torturing) and social interferences (*"I can't work or go out because of the pain"*). Where psychosocial problems are present, a team approach with a clinical psychologist or a psychiatrist may be needed.

A pain questionnaire (see Web material for Chapter 22) that the patient takes home to complete can be helpful in complex cases. It allows time for a patient to consider important aspects of their pain and to write them down. Patients can feel unsure and intimidated by dentists, physicians and psychiatrists when they ask personal questions. Therefore, some information may not be readily disclosed. For example, menopausal women are predisposed to various persistent trigeminal pain states. Although estrogens have a primary role in reproductive pathways, they also have an important role in bone metabolism and pain pathways.

Psychosocial and behavioral factors

Psychosocial and behavioral factors can trigger or maintain neuropathic orofacial pain.

Triggering factors

The onset of neuropathic orofacial pain often coincides with a stressful life event that occurred just prior to the onset of pain. Stress releases rapidly acting neurotransmitters such as epinephrine, which can amplify CNS responses and make the patient more aware of pain and other stimuli. Stressful life events that may *trigger a pain event* include:

- Death or serious injury
- Illness to a family member or friend
- Near-death experience of the patient
- Financial strain or job loss
- Marriage problems, divorce or separation
- A happy but stressful event (wedding planning)
- Legal issues
- Cultural adjustment
- Major problems with family or children.

Maintaining factors

A number of behavioral and psychological traits can result in perpetuating orofacial neuropathic pain states.

These include:

- *Persistence of stressful situations*: Psychosocial characteristics, such as being a *perfectionist* or *chronic worrier*, can play an important role in maintaining pain due to increased levels of neuropeptides including substance P.
- *Catastrophization*: Some patients with overdramatic expressive personalities can amplify pain descriptions (*"The pain is the worst anyone could possibly have!"*). Similarly, when determining the effectiveness of a pain medication, any side effects can be amplified by the patient, masking the actual benefit of the medication. These patients can have a negative outlook on *any* treatment strategy. Statements from these patients may include *"What if the medication does not work?"* or *"The next medication did not work"* or *"The last medication you gave me did not work!"*
- *Unrealistic expectations*: If patients have had pain for many years (e.g. severe pain for 20 years), they should not expect to get 100% pain relief. It is important to inform these patients that *chronic pain must be managed rather than cured*. It is rare to get a *total pain cure*.
- *Manipulation*: Patients can be manipulative and deliberately report false facts. Be observant for manipulative patients, partners or caregivers who manipulate information for personal advantage, financial gain (litigation), justification for work absences or sourcing prescription drugs.
- *Aggression*: Patients can challenge or insult the practitioner: *"So you think you can fix my pain, doctor, when everyone else has failed."*
- *Pain breakthrough*: Occasionally patients report episodes of high-intensity pain and tell you, *"Doctor, the treatment is not working anymore."* In these cases, look at recent higher levels of stress

that can explain the increased pain. Despite being anatomically remote, pathophysiological factors such as trauma, infection or surgical intervention in another area of the body can lead to increased levels of circulating pain mediators that sensitize the trigeminal nerve and increase the level of pain.

- *Drug and alcohol abuse*: Pain medication works poorly in patients who abuse drugs or alcohol.
- *Psychological distress*: When patients describe pain as *"cruel, devastating, unbearable, torturing, or punishing,"* they are indicating a high level of psychological distress. These are emotive descriptors of pain and not physiological descriptors.
- *Psychiatric issues*: *"Doctor, I see little people squeeze under the closed door, climb up the curtain next to the bed, jump onto my head, lift it off the top of my skull and press buttons in my brain to start the pain in my face…"* (actual case description).
- *Depressive illness*: Chronic pain is often associated with depression. If depression is recognized and appropriate psychological help or medication is prescribed, many patients can be relieved of this devastating condition and can cope more effectively with the pain.
- *Some physiological diseases* have multiple somatic symptoms (e.g. multiple sclerosis and systemic lupus erythematosus).

Management

Patients with complex pain problems are difficult to manage. They attempt to manipulate, are critical of previous treatment and demand that a certain treatment be started immediately. The best place for these patients is with someone else who is experienced in managing patients with complex and challenging pain conditions. It is too easy for an inexperienced but compassionate practitioner to embark on treatment that a patient demands rather than developing a sound treatment plan derived from careful diagnosis. Commencing treatment without a proper diagnosis can have unsatisfactory or even tragic outcomes for both the patient and the practitioner.

Philosophically and legally, it is far better to have a patient who dislikes you because you did not perform treatment than one who dislikes you because you performed treatment that was unnecessary, did not solve the problem and may have created an even worse one.

NOTES:

- Be vigilant in treating patients who demand analgesics or other medications, as there may be an underlying drug dependency. Patients can feign a pain problem solely to gain access to medication.
- Be sure of a diagnosis before commencing treatment for patients who:

Omit key pieces of history.

Patients who omit information may be deliberately concealing non-compliance with previous treatment advice.

Are taking large doses of analgesics or other medication.

Excessive consumption of analgesics implies two possibilities, either desperation for pain relief or an underlying addiction. It is necessary to contact a physician for assistance.

Complain of pain that crosses the midline or appears in other parts of the body.

This is a red flag in diagnosis. It is not uncommon for neuropathic pains to cross the midline and appear in other parts of the body. This is not a feature of pain of dental origin.

Arrive for diagnosis with a partner who may do most of the talking.

Some partners are controlling in a relationship, even in medical issues. This can cause undue patient stress and result in the development of stress-related illnesses or other psychologically related health problems.

Who arrive for diagnosis with a large dossier of reports and opinions from other practitioners or who are overly critical of past treatment.

This is a red flag for patient management. While detailed information is helpful, many patients who arrive with comprehensive notes can be fixated on the problem and what *they* consider the cause, rather than listening to an alternative diagnosis.

Insist that a specific form of treatment be undertaken and in a specified manner.

With the availability of the Internet, patients are all too willing to be "Dr. Google." This is a red flag for the practitioner and heightens the need to be sure of a diagnosis before any treatment is undertaken, as the patient is likely to be non-compliant.

Are non-compliant with treatment recommendations.

Patients are ultimately responsible for following sound health advice.

Questions to ask if trigeminal neuropathic facial pain is suspected

What sort of pain are you having?

Neuropathic pain is constant, aching, burning or throbbing.

What do you feel caused the pain?

Patients often claim onset of pain following dental treatment.

Was there a very stressful life event that occurred just prior to the onset of your pain?

Neuropathic orofacial pain is often precipitated by a stressful life event.

Are you under any stress right now?

Stress can amplify the intensity of pain. It is important to identify stress and explain the direct relationship between high stress and increasingly severe pain.

Is the stressful situation going on now with no end in sight, or do you see an end to it?

Ask the patient if there is ongoing stress involving finances, health or family/marital relationships. It is difficult for the person to improve while there is persistent stress.

Does medication relieve the pain?

Commonly prescribed analgesics such as ibuprofen, codeine/paracetamol (Panadeine Forte®) or Tylenol #3® (acetaminophen/codeine) cause only a slight reduction or no change in pain intensity.

Is the pain spreading to other areas?

Neuropathic pain spreads and can cross the midline due to CNS maladaptive neuroplasticity.

Does local anesthesia stop the pain?

A partial or poor response to local anesthesia is due to CNS activation and alteration in the calcium ion channels.

Do you suffer from headaches, neck aches or jaw muscle pain?

Seventy percent of patients with neuropathic pain develop temporomandibular disorders.

Do you notice episodes of swelling in the cheek?

Sixty to seventy percent of patients with trigeminal neuropathic pain develop sympathetic nervous system hyperfunction.

Presentation and confirmation tests

- Normal clinical and radiographic appearance, yet there is long-term pain.
- Pain descriptors include *constant, aching, burning, throbbing* and *sharp*.
- Referral to an experienced practitioner for a correct diagnosis.
- Lignocaine IV infusion for neuropathic pain to assess the sodium channel contribution to neuropathic pain. If a positive response (reduced pain) is recorded, a trial of mexiletine can be considered.
- Phentolamine infusion for sympathetically maintained pain. A positive response (reduced pain)[237] suggests sympathetic ganglion blockade. Bupivacaine or guanethidine may be helpful.
- Good response of neuropathic pain to antidepressants and anticonvulsants.

Treatment considerations

As treatment of patients with neuropathic pain is not always easy, a three-pronged approach is necessary: reassurance, medication and psychological management.

Reassurance

- Reassure the patient that their pain is real and give a diagnosis.
- Reduce uncertainty and fear by providing a clear explanation of the nature of the pain.
- Listen without being judgmental.
  Patients may criticize other health professionals. Some patients are angry at physicians or dentists who they believe have failed them by not relieving their pain.

- Offer *referral for pain management* and explain the reason that complex pain requires a multidisciplinary approach involving dental, medical, physical and psychological care.

Medication

For neuropathic pain, typically the first line of anti-neuropathic agents are tricyclic antidepressants (TCAs) and anticonvulsants. The inclusion of medication for orofacial pain management should be under the general supervision of the general medical practitioner. An important consideration is the potential for side effects and drug interactions from the chronic pain medications. Dry mouth, drowsiness, weight gain, mood change and gastrointestinal disturbance occur with TCAs. Drowsiness and CNS side effects can occur with anticonvulsants. The importance of the appropriate dental management of patients with drug-induced xerostomia cannot be overemphasized:

- Application of topical capsaicin (0.025–0.075%) to painful mucosa for 5 to 10 minutes, twice a day, for 6 weeks can be helpful. Pre-treat the area with topical anesthetic mouthwash to prevent discomfort when applying the capsaicin. This strategy can be very effective if used in the first few months after the onset of neuropathic pain.[237]
- Tricyclic antidepressants, including prothiaden, amitriptyline or nortriptyline, titrated to an analgesic dose if there is burning pain (usually 25 mg in the evening, but may need to increase dosage to 75 mg over 3 weeks). Maintain medication for 18 months.[238]
- Anticonvulsants such as pregabalin, gabapentin, carbamazepine or sodium valproate, titrated if there is sharp, shooting pain.[230,240]
- Where pain involves aching/burning (C fiber pain) and sharp/shooting (A-delta fiber pain), then polypharmacy is indicated using tricyclic antidepressants and anticonvulsants.
- Other medications used by pain specialists for neuropathic pain include opioid drugs (morphine), mexiletine (cardiac anti-arrythmic), palmitoylethanolamide (natural compound from egg yolk and peanut oil) and 6-gingerol (from fresh ginger).
- Autologous stem cell therapy has recently been shown to be safe and effective for treating neuropathic pain.[241]

Psychological treatment

Psychological relaxation exercises and cognitive behavioral techniques are used to reduce background stress and anxiety. This can be particularly helpful when the patient describes the pain using emotional or affective terms such as *maddening, punishing, excruciating, terrifying* or *cruel*.

Chapter 23

Referral Strategies for Orofacial Pain Cases

E. Russell Vickers and Alex J. Moule

Introduction

On occasion, it is necessary to refer a patient to a dental or medical specialist for diagnosis, treatment or management of orofacial pain.[242] A knowledgeable and mature clinician refers patients for improved care if their management proves unsuccessful. This is one of the highest principles in clinical practice.

Referral patterns vary from practitioner to practitioner. Nevertheless, referrals cannot, or do not, take place if the identity of an appropriate medical or dental specialist is not known. It is good practice policy, therefore, to have contact information at hand for each dental or medical specialty, so that referrals can be made seamlessly when the need arises. There is also a definite advantage if a practitioner has already considered the possibility of referring a difficult patient, and has the appropriate information available before a patient returns repeatedly for weeks or months still complaining of persistent pain. Multiple failed visits to relieve pain leads to a loss of a patient's confidence in their health provider.

Before referral, obtain as much information as possible on the relevant history of the problem, carrying out all normal testing procedures and radiographic examinations that will assist in the diagnosis by the specialist. The specialist can order more important tests such as specific radiographs, MRI, CT or CBCT imaging, bone scans and blood tests as necessary. Medico-legally, phone calls and referral letters to specialists should be recorded and archived. This confirms appropriate and timely care.

Coordinating with the general medical practitioner

With complex pain patients, a telephone call to the patient's General Medical Practitioner (GMP) or other treating clinicians is imperative. Thus, the patient is not treated in isolation and various treatment regimens can be coordinated. Privacy issues need to be recognized and addressed. A patient's permission is necessary before consulting with another clinician. Nevertheless, if a patient wants to be helped, they should agree to have their pain problems discussed with fellow clinicians. While consultations with other caregivers are an important part of assessing a patient with orofacial pain, care should be taken in reaching an independent diagnosis and not to be influenced by the opinions of others.

As mentioned in other chapters in this book, persistent orofacial pain is a bio-psychosocial problem for which a patient's management may need to be coordinated with a medical general practitioner (GMP), and medical and dental specialists. Where appropriate, the GMP may involve a neurologist for trigeminal nerve conditions with origins in the CNS, a musculoskeletal physician where there is widespread myofascial pain that may include the dental component of temporomandibular disorders, or other specialists. Furthermore, where there are pre-existing psychological problems or obvious negative psychological changes due to pain, inclusion of a clinical psychologist or psychiatrist is necessary.

Indications of urgent referral

Orofacial pain encompasses a wide range of pathological conditions. In most cases, the cause of the pain can be diagnosed and controlled by the general dental clinician. Referral is necessary, however, in circumstances where the clinician is uncertain about the origin of the pain, where there is a need for urgent diagnosis and treatment, or where chronic or persistent pain conditions have to be *managed* rather than treated.

Urgent referral is necessary if a patient has intractable pain that cannot be managed by the clinician, or

Diagnosing Dental and Orofacial Pain: A Clinical Manual, First Edition. Edited by Alex J. Moule and M. Lamar Hicks.
© 2017 John Wiley & Sons, Ltd. Published 2017 by John Wiley & Sons, Ltd.
Companion website: www.wiley.com/go/moule/dental_and_orofacial_pain

if the severe orofacial pain is suspected to be of non-dental origin, including malignancy. Indications for conditions that require urgent referral include:

- *Facial pain in the temple suggesting cranial (temporal) arteritis.* This is inflammation and pain originating in the temporal artery, which may occur after high doses of antibiotics. Diagnosis is by the history and an erythrocyte sedimentation rate (ESR) blood test. Treatment is with high doses of corticosteroids to prevent an infarct in the involved cranial nerves, which can lead to permanent blindness if the optic nerve is involved.
- *Pain in the mastoid region indicating mastoiditis.* A middle ear infection may spread to the mastoid process behind the ear causing severe pain, redness and swelling in the region. Treatment is with antibiotics.
- *Rapid swelling with pain suggesting infection of a tissue plane and potential cellulitis.* Dental infection may spread along tissue planes causing rapid involvement of the submandibular, buccal or lateral pharyngeal fascial spaces, potentially causing airway restriction and death. Treatment is immediate hospitalization and aggressive treatment with IV antibiotics and drainage.
- *Increasing facial numbness, loss of taste or paresis suggesting CNS tumor.* Tumors of the cranial nerves (CNs) can occur causing facial numbness (trigeminal nerve, CN V), facial palsy/paresis (facial nerve, CN VII) and loss of taste (glossopharyngeal nerve, CN IX) from pressure on the nerve caused by growth of a benign tumor or nerve destruction by direct invasion of the nerve by a malignant tumor.
- *Sharp, shooting needle-like pain* suggesting trigeminal neuralgia (face), glossopharyngeal neuralgia (tongue/throat on swallowing) or multiple sclerosis, in which the A-delta pain nerve fibers become demyelinated causing a trigeminal neuralgia or spontaneous neuralgic pain.
- *Very severe headache of rapidly increasing severity* suggesting intracranial hemorrhage (aneurysm). This is life threatening and requires emergency admission to hospital and MRI.
- *Persistent pain still present 4–6 weeks after a dental procedure* that eliminated a different pain (e.g. following a tooth extraction or endodontic treatment). This scenario is suggestive of neurogenic inflammation, which requires definitive diagnosis and treatment. Referral to an endodontist or oral surgeon for management of this condition should be considered.

Referral for pain diagnosis and management

There are occasions where it is necessary to refer a patient for *pain management*, rather than *total pain relief* or a cure. Many patients with chronic intractable pain require referral to pain clinics or to clinicians skilled in the pharmacological and psychological management of patients with chronic orofacial pain. Early referral for pain management is of prime importance, with far better outcomes realized before chronic pain disease states affect other systems such as the immune, neuronal and muscular systems. Delaying referral increases psychological distress and suffering.

Most countries have dental and medical pain specialists. In addition, there are multidisciplinary pain clinics at major teaching hospitals and national professional pain organizations such as the International Association for the Study of Pain which have affiliated national chapters (see www.iasp-pain.org).

Pain clinics have specialists in anesthesia, neurology, psychiatry, rheumatology, psychology, physiotherapy and dentistry. A pain clinic provides a detailed and coordinated approach to *pain management* (not pain cure). It is important that the dentist explains to the patient why they are being referred. That explanation should include that chronic pain, irrespective of location, is a medical disease state that is similar to diabetes or cardiovascular disease, and that without proper treatment the disease progresses.

NOTE: It is important to be honest with the patient when referring to a specialist or pain clinic for pain management. It may be easier to make a statement such as:

I have not been able to help you.
You are probably always going to have some pain.
Can we see if we can find someone who can help you manage the pain better?

Useful questions to consider when assessing whether to refer a patient

How does the pain affect their daily routine?
Be careful diagnosing pain in patients who describe severe pain, but who seem to be able to perform their usual daily routine without inconvenience.
Is there a relationship between pressure or stress and the intensity of the pain?
Pain may wax and wane. Whether the patient's pain is prominent, in the background or absent may reflect or depend on the emotional state of the patient at the time of presentation.
Have you had pain for more than three months?
By definition, chronic pain is pain of three or more month. In most cases, referral is in the patient's best interest.
Is the intensity of the pain the same or getting worse since you first noticed it?
Chronic pain is recognized as a disease process and worsens with time.

Is the pain spreading to other areas?

This suggests maladaptive neuroplasticity of other nerves, and interneuron activation to cause muscle spasm and sympathetic nervous system activation.

Does the pain cause you distress or suffering?

A practitioner must be aware of negative psychological and social changes that require referral of the patient to a clinical psychologist.

Does the pain disturb your sleep frequently?

An altered sleep pattern will increase pain. Patients with chronic pain often have disturbed sleep patterns. Consultation with a physician is required.

Does the pain cause you to sometimes feel despair, panic, or sad and depressed?

A patient's affirmative response strongly suggests a referral to a psychiatrist. Constant high-intensity pain can cause desperate attempts by the patient to remove it or end the pain by desperate actions such as suicide.

Do you believe that your current pain medication is inadequate?

The need to increase the dose of pain medication can indicate the development of tolerance to the drug. Thus, to gain the desired effect from the drug, there is a need to increase the dosage or switch to an alternative medication. It can also mean multiple, but different, concurrent pain states have developed. An example is neuropathic pain with myofascial pain.

Have you consulted many other health professionals for your pain?

This question implies there is still "no diagnosis." Referral to a pain specialist will provide an accurate diagnosis and prevent unnecessary procedures and incorrect treatment.

How can I help you manage the pain a little better?

This emphasis on *pain management* is particularly important when a referral to a psychologist or to a psychiatrist is contemplated.

References

Chapter 2

1. Stein, P.S., Aalboe, J.A., Savage, M.W. & Scott, A.M. (2014). Strategies for communicating with older dental patients. *J Am Dent Assoc.*, **145(2)**, 159–164.
2. Wolvin, A.D. (2003). The medical patient as listener: expanding the health literacy model. Paper presented to International Listening Association Annual Conference 2003. Available at: http://www.listen.org/Listening_Resources [accessed 28 July 2014].
3. Sondell, K. & Soderfeldt, B. (1997). Dentist-patient communication: a review of relevant models. *Acta Odontol Scand.*, **55(2)**,116–126.
4. Rozier, R.G., Horowitz, A.M. & Podschun, G. (2011). Dentist-patient communication techniques used in the United States: the results of a national survey. *J Am Dent Assoc.*, **142(5)**, 518–530.
5. Travaline, J.M., Ruchinskas, R. & D'Alonzo. G.E., Jr. (2005). Patient-physician communication: why and how. *J Am Osteopath Assoc.*, **105(1)**, 13–18.
6. Wolvin, A.D. (2010). *Listening and Human Communication in the 21st Century*. Chichester, UK; Malden, MA: Wiley-Blackwell. xii, 299 p.
7. Brownell, J. (2010). *Listening*. Boston: Allyn & Bacon.
8. Marvel, M.K., Epstein, R.M., Flowers, K. & Beckman, H.B. (1999). Soliciting the patient's agenda: have we improved? *JAMA*, **281(3)**, 283–287.
9. Mehrabian, A. (1971). *Silent Messages*. Belmont, CA: Wadsworth Publishing Co., viii, 152 p.
10. Mehrabian, A. (1981). *Silent Messages: Implicit Communication of Emotions and Attitudes*. 2d edn. Belmont, CA: Wadsworth Publishing Co., ix, 196 p.

Chapter 3

11. Merskey, H. (1994). Logic, truth and language in concepts of pain. *Qual Life Res.*, **3(1)**, S69–S76.
12. Zakrzewska, J.M. (1996). Assessment of a patient with orofacial pain. *Prime Dent Care*, **3(2)**, 57–60.
13. Classification and diagnostic criteria for headache disorders, cranial neuralgias and facial pain. (1988). Headache Classification Committee of the International Headache Society. *Cephalalgia*, **8(7)**, 1–96.
14. Zakrzewska, J.M. (2013). Differential diagnosis of facial pain and guidelines for management. *Br J Anaesth.*, **111(1)**, 95–104.

15. Figdor, D. (1994). Aspects of dentinal and pulpal pain. Pain of dentinal and pulpal origin – a review for the clinician. *Ann R Australas Coll Dent Surg.*, **12**, 131–142.
16. Felix, D.H., Luker, J. & Scully, C. (2012). Oral medicine. 2: Ulcers: serious ulcers. *Dent Update*, **39(8)**, 594–598.
17. Felix, D.H., Luker, J. & Scully, C. (2012). Oral medicine. 1: Ulcers: aphthous and other common ulcers. *Dent Update*, **39(7)**, 513–516, 8–9.
18. Felix, D.H., Luker, J. & Scully, C. (2012). Oral medicine. 3: Ulcers: cancer. *Dent Update*, **39(9)**, 664–668, 70.
19. Schifter, M., Yeoh, S.C., Coleman, H. & Georgiou, A. (2010). Oral mucosal diseases: the inflammatory dermatoses. *Aust Dent J.*, **55(l)**, 23–38.
20. Manfredini, D., Guarda-Nardini, L., Winocur, E., Piccotti, F., Ahlberg, J. & Lobbezoo, F. (2011). Research diagnostic criteria for temporomandibular disorders: a systematic review of axis I epidemiologic findings. *Oral Surg Oral Med Oral Pathol Oral Radiol Endod.*, **112(4)**, 453–462.
21. Simons, D.G., Travell, J.G. & Simons, L.S. (1999). *Travell & Simons' Myofascial Pain and Dysfunction: The Trigger Point Manual*. 2nd edn. Baltimore, MD: Williams & Wilkins.
22. Okeson, J.P. (2013). *Management of Temporomandibular Disorders and Occlusion*. 7th edn. St. Louis, MO: Mosby Elsvier Ltd, xiv, 488 p.
23. Biondi, D.M. (2005). Cervicogenic headache: a review of diagnostic and treatment strategies. *J Am Osteopath Assoc.*, **105(4 Suppl 2)**, 16S–22S.
24. Okeson, J.P. (2014). *Bell's Oral and Facial Pain*, 7th edn. Chicago, IL: Quintessence Publishing Co. Inc.
25. Ingle, J.I., Bakland, L.K., Baumgartner, J.C. & Ingle, J.I. (2008). *Ovid Technologies Inc. Ingle's Endodontics*, 6th edn. Hamilton, ON; Lewiston, NY: BC Decker, xxv, 1555 p.
26. Patel, N.A. & Ferguson, B.J. (2012). Odontogenic sinusitis: an ancient but under-appreciated cause of maxillary sinusitis. *Curr opinions otol head neck surg.*, **20(1)**, 24–28.
27. Binder, D.K., Sonne, D.C. & Fischbein, N.J. (2010). Cranial nerves anatomy, pathology, imaging. New York: Thieme. Available at: http://dx.doi.org/ 10.1055/b-002-74280.
28. Sulfaro, M.A. & Gobetti. J.P. (1995). Occipital neuralgia manifesting as orofacial pain. *Oral Surg Oral Med Oral Pathol Oral Radiol Endod.* 80(6), 751–755.
29. Nanci. A. & Ten Cate. A.R. (2013). *Ten Cate's Oral Histology: Development, Structure and Function*, 8th edn. St Louis, MO: Elsevier, xiii, 379 p.
30. Wilson, K.F., Meier, J.D. & Ward, P.D. (2014). Salivary gland disorders. *Am Fam Physician*, **89(11)**, 882–888.
31. Matharu, M. (2010). Cluster headache. *BMJ Clin Evid.*

32. Kawasaki, A. & Purvin, V. (2009). Giant cell arteritis: an updated review. *Acta Ophthalmol.*, **87(1)**, 13–32.

33. Schievink, W.I. (2001). Spontaneous dissection of the carotid and vertebral arteries. *N Engl J Med.*, **344(12)**, 898–906.

34. Thanvi, B., Munshi, S.K., Dawson, S.L. & Robinson, T.G. (2005). Carotid and vertebral artery dissection syndromes. *Postgrad Med J.*, **81(956)**, 383–388.

35. Balasubramaniam, R., Kuperstein, A.S. & Stoopler, E.T. (2014). Update on oral herpes virus infections. *Dent Clin North Am.*, **58(2)**, 265–280.

36. Woo, S.B. & Challacombe, S.J. (2007). Management of recurrent oral herpes simplex infections. *Oral Surg Oral Med Oral Pathol Oral Radiol Endod.*, **103 (Suppl** S12), e1–e8.

37. Dworkin, R.H., Gnann, J.W., Jr., Oaklander, A.L., Raja, S.N., Schmader, K.E. & Whitley, R.J. (2008). Diagnosis and assessment of pain associated with herpes zoster and post-herpetic neuralgia. *J Pain*, **9(1 Suppl 1)**, S37–S44.

38. Teodoro, F.C., Tronco, M.F., Jr., Zampronio, A.R., Martini, A.C., Rae, G.A. & Chichorro, J.G. (2013). Peripheral substance P and neurokinin-1 receptors have a role in inflammatory and neuropathic orofacial pain models. *Neuropeptides*, **47(3)**, 199–206.

39. Bartolini, A., Di Cesare Mannelli, L. & Ghelardini, C. (2011). Analgesic and antineuropathic drugs acting through central cholinergic mechanisms. *Recent Pat CNS Drug Discov.*, **6(2)**, 119–140.

40. Ren, K. & Dubner, R. (1999). Central nervous system plasticity and persistent pain. *J Orofac Pain*, **13(3)**, 155–163; discussion 64–71.

41. Aggarwal, V.R., McBeth, J., Zakrzewska, J.M., Lunt, M. & Macfarlane, G.J. (2006). The epidemiology of chronic syndromes that are frequently unexplained: do they have common associated factors? *Int J Epidemiol.*, **35(2)**, 468–476.

42. Okeson, J.P. & Bell, W.E. (2005). *Bell's Orofacial Pains: The Clinical Management of Orofacial Pain*, 6th edn. Chicago, IL: Quintessence Publishing Co. Inc., xvi, 567 p.

43. Lynch, K.M. & Brett, F. (2012). Headaches that kill: a retrospective study of incidence, etiology and clinical features in cases of sudden death. *Cephalalgia*, **32(13)**, 972–978.

44. Dworkin, S.I., Porrino, L.J. & Smith, J.E. (1992). Importance of behavioral controls in the analysis of ongoing events. *NIDA Res Monogr.*, **124**, 173–188.

45. Gatchel, R.J., Garofalo, J.P., Ellis, E. & Holt, C. (1996). Major psychological disorders in acute and chronic TMD: an initial examination. *J Am Dent Assoc.*, **127(9)**, 1365–1370, 72, 74.

Chapter 4

46. Okeson, J.P. & Bell, W.E. (2005). *Bell's Orofacial Pains: The Clinical Management of Orofacial Pain*, 6th edn. Chicago, IL: Quintessence Publishing Co. Inc.

47. Beckman, H.B. & Frankel, R.M. (1984). The effect of physician behavior on the collection of data. *Ann Intern Med.*, **101(5)**, 692–696.

48. Ryle, J.A. (1936). *The Natural History of Disease.* London: Oxford University Press.

49. Dyche, L. & Swiderski, D. (2005). The effect of physician solicitation approaches on ability to identify patient concerns. *J Gen Intern Med.*, **20(3)**, 267–270.

50. Blau, J.N. (1982). How to take a history of head or facial pain. *Br Med J.*, **285(6350)**, 1249–1251.

51. Kent, G. (1984). Anxiety, pain and type of dental procedure. *Behav Res Ther.*, **22(5)**, 465–469.

Chapter 5

52. Apkarian, A.V., Hashmi, J.A. & Baliki, M.N. (2011). Pain and the brain: specificity and plasticity of the brain in clinical chronic pain. *Pain*, **152(3 Suppl)**, S49–S64.

53. Lance, J.W. *Mechanism and Management of Headache*, 5th edn.

54. Melzack, R. (1975). The *McGill Pain Questionnaire*: major properties and scoring methods. *Pain*, **1(3)**, 277–299.

55. Grushka, M. & Sessle, B.J. (1984). Applicability of the McGill Pain Questionnaire to the differentiation of "toothache" pain. *Pain*, **19(1)**, 49–57.

56. Okeson, J.P. & Bell, W.E. (2005). *Bell's Orofacial Pains: The Clinical Management of Orofacial Pain*, 6th edn. Chicago, IL: Quintessence Publishing Co. Inc., pp. 147–148.

Chapter 6

57. Lance, J.W. & Goadsby, P.J. (2005). *Mechanism and Management of Headache*, 7th edn. Philadelphia: Elsevier; Butterworth, Heinemann; xx, 392 p.

58. Lynch, K.M. & Brett, F. (2012). Headaches that kill: a retrospective study of incidence, etiology and clinical features in cases of sudden death. *Cephalalgia*, **32(13)**, 972–978.

59. Moule, A.J. (2004). *Orofacial Pain – What the Patient is telling You.* Brighton Qld: Knowledge Books and Software, ix, 124 p.

Chapter 8

60. Su, N., Ching, V. & Grushka, M. Taste disorders: a review. *J Can Dent Assoc.*, **79**, d86.

61. Lyons, K.M., Rodda, J.C. & Hood, J.A. (1999). Barodontalgia: a review, and the influence of simulated diving on microleakage and on the retention of full cast crowns. *Mil Med.*, **164(3)**, 221–227.

62. Rauch, J.W. (1985). Barodontalgia – dental pain related to ambient pressure change. *Gen Dent.*, **33(4)**, 313–315.

Chapter 9

63. Okeson, J.P. & Bell, W.E. (2005). *Bell's Orofacial Pains: The Clinical Management of Orofacial Pain*, 6th edn. Chicago, IL: Quintessence Publishing Co Inc., p. 142.

64. Lynch, K.M. & Brett, F. (2012). Headaches that kill: a retrospective study of incidence, etiology and clinical features in cases of sudden death. *Cephalalgia*. **32(13)**, 972–978.

Chapter 10

65. Okeson, J.P. & Bell, W.E. (2005). *Bell's Orofacial Pains: The Clinical Management of Orofacial Pain*, 6th edn. Chicago, IL: Quintessence Publishing Co. Inc., p. 318.

Chapter 11

66. Hargreaves. K. & Cohen. S. (2011). *Pathways of Pulp*, 10th edn. St Louis, MO: Mosby Elsevier, Ltd, pp. 16–17.

67. Mejare, I.A., Axelsson, S., Davidson, T., Frisk, F., Hakeberg, M., et al. (2012). Diagnosis of the condition of the dental pulp: a systematic review. *Int Endod J.*, **45(7)**, 597–613.

68. McCarthy, P.J., McClanahan, S., Hodges, J. & Bowles, W.R. (2010). Frequency of localization of the painful tooth by patients presenting for an endodontic emergency. *J Endod.*, **36(5)**, 801–805.

69. Keiser, K. & Hargreaves, K.M. (2002). Building effective strategies for the management of endodontic pain. *Endodontic Topics*, **3(1)**, 93–105.

70. Van Hassel, H.J. & Harrington, G.W. (1969). Localization of pulpal sensation. *Oral Surg Oral Med Oral Pathol.*, **28(5)**, 753–760.

71. Falace, D.A., Reid, K. & Rayens, M.K. (1996). The influence of deep (odontogenic) pain intensity, quality, and duration on the incidence and characteristics of referred orofacial pain. *J Orofac Pain*, **10(3)**, 232–239.

72. Ricucci, D., Pascon, E.A., Ford, T.R. & Langeland, K. (2006). Epithelium and bacteria in periapical lesions. *Oral Surg Oral Med Oral Pathol Oral Radiol Endod.*, **101(2)**, 239–249.

73. Jafarzadeh, H. & Abbott, P.V. Review of pulp sensibility tests. Part II: electric pulp tests and test cavities. *Int Endod J.*, **43(11)**, 945–958.

74. Nusstein, J.M. & Beck, M. (2003). Comparison of preoperative pain and medication use in emergency patients presenting with irreversible pulpitis or teeth with necrotic pulps. *Oral Surg Oral Med Oral Pathol Oral Radiol Endod.*, **96(2)**, 207–214.

75. Read, J.K., McClanahan, S.B., Khan, A.A., Lunos, S. & Bowles, W.R. (2014). Effect of Ibuprofen on masking endodontic diagnosis. *J Endod.* **40(8)**, 1058–1062.

76. Khan, A.A., Owatz, C.B., Schindler, W.G., Schwartz, S.A., Keiser, K. & Hargreaves, K.M. (2007). Measurement of mechanical allodynia and local anesthetic efficacy in patients with irreversible pulpitis and acute periradicular periodontitis. *J Endod.*, **33(7)**, 796–799.

77. Boucher, Y., Sobel, M. & Sauveur, G. (2000). Persistent pain related to root canal filling and apical fenestration: a case report. *J Endod.*, **26(4)**, 242–244.

78. Moule, A.J. & Kahler, B. (1999). Diagnosis and management of teeth with vertical root fractures. *Aust Dent J.*, **44(2)**, 75–87.

79. Pigg, M., List, T., Petersson, K., Lindh, C. & Petersson, A. (2011). Diagnostic yield of conventional radiographic and cone-beam computed tomographic images in patients with atypical odontalgia. *Int Endod J.*, **44(12)**, 1092–1101.

80. Abella, F., Patel, S., Duran-Sindreu, F., Mercade, M., Bueno, R. & Roig, M. (2014). An evaluation of the periapical status of teeth with necrotic pulps using periapical radiography and cone-beam computed tomography. *Int Endod J.*, **47(4)**, 387–396.

81. Okeson, J.P. (2005). *Principles of Pain Diagnosis. Bell's Orofacial Pains*, 6th edn. Chicago, IL: Quintessence Publishing Co, Inc., pp. 183–184.

82. Okeson, J.P. (2005). *Neuropathic Pains. Bell's Orofacial Pains*, 6th edn. Chicago, IL: Quintessence Publishing Co. Inc., pp. 457–459.

83. Berman, L. & Hartwell, G. (2011). Diagnosis. In: *Cohen's Pathways of the Pulp*, 10th edn (eds K. Hargreaves and S. Cohen), St Louis, MO: Mosby Elsevier, Ltd, p. 19.

84. Marotti, J., Heger, S., Tinschert, J., Tortamano, P., Chuembou, F., *et al.* (2013). Recent advances of ultrasound imaging in dentistry – a review of the literature. *Oral Surg Oral Med Oral Path Oral Rad.*, **115(6)**, 819–832.

Chapter 12

85. Zakrzewska, J.M. (2013). Differential diagnosis of facial pain and guidelines for management. *Br J Anaesth.*, **111(1)**, 95–104.

86. Figdor, D. (1994). Aspects of dentinal and pulpal pain. Pain of dentinal and pulpal origin – a review for the clinician. *Ann R Australas Coll Dent Surg.*, **12**, 131–142.

87. Seltzer, S., Bender, I.B. & Ziontz, M. (1963). The dynamics of pulp inflammation: correlations between diagnostic data and actual histologic findings in the pulp. *Oral Surg Oral Med Oral Pathol.*, **16**, 969–977.

88. Ricucci, D., Loghin, S. & Siqueira, J.F., Jr. (2014). Correlation between clinical and histologic pulp diagnoses. *J Endod.*, **40(12)**, 1932–1939.

89. AAE Consensus Conference Recommended Diagnostic Terminology: American Association of Endodontists (2009). [06-08-2014]. Available at: http://www.aae.org/uploadedfiles/publications_and_research/newsletters/endodontics_colleagues_for_excellence_newsletter/aaeconsensusconferencerecommendeddiagnostictermi-nology.pdf

90. Michaelson, P.L. & Holland, G.R. (2002). Is pulpitis painful? *Int Endod J.*, **35(10)**, 829–832.

91. Abou-Rass, M. (1982). The stressed pulp condition: an endodontic-restorative diagnostic concept. *J Prosthet Dent.*, **48(3)**, 264–267.

92. Fouad, A.F. & Levin, L. (2011). Pulpal reaction to caries and dental procedures. In: *Cohen's Pathways of the Pulp*, 10th edn (eds K. Hargreaves & L. Berman), St Louis, MO: Mosby Elsevier Ltd, pp. 504–506.

93. Epstein, O., Perkins, G.D. & Cookson, J. (2008). *Consultation, Medical History and Record Taking*, 4th edn. St Louis, MO: Mosby Elsevier Ltd, pp. 1–19.

94. Hargreaves, K. & Cohen, S. (2011). *Cohen's Pathways of the Pulp*, 10th edn. St Louis, MO: Mosby Elsevier, Ltd.

95. Siqueira, J.F., Jr. (2011). *Treatment of Endodontic Infections*, 1st edn. Chicago, IL: Quintessence Publishing Co, Inc.

96. Okeson, J.P. (2005). The processing of pain at the brainstem level. In: *Bell's Orofacial Pains*, 6th edn. Chicago, IL: Quintessence Publishing Co. Inc., pp. 65–73.

97. Broton, J.G., Hu, J.W. & Sessle, B.J. (1988). Effects of temporomandibular joint stimulation on nociceptive and nonnociceptive neurons of the cat's trigeminal subnucleus caudalis (medullary dorsal horn). *J Neurophysiol.*, **59(5)**, 1575–1589.

98. Mattscheck, D., Law, A.S. & Nixdorf, D.R. (2011). Diagnosis of nonodontogenic toothache. In: *Cohen's Pathways of the Pulp*, 10th edn. (eds K. Hargreaves & S. Cohen), St Louis, MO: Mosby Elsevier, Ltd, pp. 50–55.

99. Rocha, A.P., Kraychete, D.C., Lemonica, L., de Carvalho, L.R., de Barros, G.A., *et al.* (2007). Pain: current aspects on peripheral and central sensitization. *Rev Bras Anestesiol.*, **57(1)**, 94–105.

Chapter 13

100. Kim, S.Y., Kim, S.H., Cho, S.B., Lee, G.O. & Yang, S.E. (2013). Different treatment protocols for different pulpal and periapical diagnoses of 72 cracked teeth. *J Endod.*, **39(4)**, 449–452.

101. Cameron, C.E. (1964). *Cracked-tooth syndrome. J Am Dent Assoc.*, **68**, 405–411.

102. Homewood, C.I. (1998). Cracked tooth syndrome – incidence, clinical findings and treatment. *Aust Dent J.*, **43(4)**, 217–222.

103. Cavel, W.T., Kelsey, W.P. & Blankenau, R.J. (1985). An *in vivo* study of cuspal fracture. *J Prosthet Dent.*, **53(1)**, 38–42.

104. Braly, B.V. & Maxwell, E.H. (1981). Potential for tooth fracture in restorative dentistry. *J Prosthet Dent.*, **45(4):** 411–414.

105. Kahler, B., Moule, A. & Stenzel, D. (2000). Bacterial contamination of cracks in symptomatic vital teeth. *Aust Endodon J.*, **26(3)**, 115–118.

106. Brannstrom, M. (1986). The hydrodynamic theory of dentinal pain: sensation in preparations, caries, and the dentinal crack syndrome. *J Endod.*, **12(10)**, 453–457.

107. Tennert, C., Eismann, M., Goetz, F., Woelber, J.P., Hellwig, E. & Polydorou, O. (2015). A temporary filling material used for coronal sealing during endodontic treatment may cause tooth fractures in large Class II cavities *in vitro*. *Int Endod J.*, **48(1)**, 84–88.

108. Moule, A.J. & Kahler, B. (1999). Diagnosis and management of teeth with vertical root fractures. *Aust Dent J.*, **44(2)**, 75–87.

109. Berman, L.H. & Kuttler, S. (2010). Fracture necrosis: diagnosis, prognosis assessment and treatment recommendations. *J Endod.*, **36(3)**, 442–446.

110. Yang, S.F., Rivera, E.M. & Walton, R.E. (1995). Vertical root fracture in nonendodontically treated teeth. *J Endod.*, **21(6)**, 337–339.

111. Yeh, C.J. (1997). Fatigue root fracture: a spontaneous root fracture in non-endodontically treated teeth. *Br Dent J.*, **182(7)**, 261–266.

112. Signore, A., Benedicenti, S., Covani, U. & Ravera, G. (2007). A 4- to 6-year retrospective clinical study of cracked teeth restored with bonded indirect resin composite onlays. *Int J Prosthodont.*, **20(6)**, 609–616.

113. Opdam, N.J., Roeters, J.J., Loomans, B.A. & Bronkhorst, E.M. (2008). Seven-year clinical evaluation of painful cracked teeth restored with a direct composite restoration. *J Endod.*, **34(7)**, 808–811.

114. Banerji, S., Mehta, S.B. & Millar, B.J. (2010). Cracked tooth syndrome. Part 2: Restorative options for the management of cracked tooth syndrome. *Br Dent J.*, **208(11)**, 503–514.

115. Tan, L., Chen, N.N., Pyoon, C.Y. & Wong, H.B. (2006). Survival of root filled cracked teeth in a tertiary institution. *Int Endo J.*, **39**, 886–889.

116. Seo, D.,Yi, Y., Shin, S. & Park, J. (2012). Analysis of factors associated with cracked teeth. *J Endod.*, **38(3)**, 288–292.

117. Bader, J.D., Shugars, D.A. & Sturdevant, J.R. (2004). Consequences of posterior cusp fracture. *Gen Dent.*, **52(2)**, 128–131.

118. Zimet, P.O. (1998). Cracked tooth syndrome. *Aust Endod J.*, **24(1)**, 33–37.

Chapter 14

119. Manfredini, D., Guarda-Nardini, L., Winocur, E., Piccotti, F., Ahlberg, J. & Lobbezoo, F. (2011). Research diagnostic criteria for temporomandibular disorders: a systematic review of axis I epidemiologic findings. *Oral Surg Oral Med Oral Path Oral Rad Endod.*, **112(4)**, 453–462.

120. Simons, D.G., Travell, J.G. & Simons, L.S. (1999). *Travell and Simons' Myofascial Pain and Dysfunction: The Trigger Point Manual*, 2nd edn. Baltimore: Williams & Wilkins.

121. Schiffman, E., Ohrbach, R., Truelove, E., Look, J., Anderson, G., *et al.* (2014). Diagnostic Criteria for Temporomandibular Disorders (DC/TMD) for Clinical and Research Applications: recommendations of the International RDC/TMD Consortium Network* and Orofacial Pain Special Interest Groupdagger. *J Oral Fac Pain Headache*, **28(1)**, 6–27.

122. Okeson, J.P. (2013). *Management of Temporomandibular Disorders and Occlusion*, 7th edn. St. Louis, MO: Elsevier Mosby Ltd, ix, p. 488.

123. Klineberg, I. & Jagger, R.G. (2004). *Occlusion and Clinical Practice: An Evidence-based Approach*. Edinburgh: Wright, xi, 145 p.

124. Gustin, S.M., Peck, C.C., Cheney, L.B., Macey, P.M., Murray, G.M. & Henderson, L.A. (2012). Pain and plasticity: is chronic pain always associated with somatosensory cortex activity and reorganization? *J Neurosci.*, **32(43)**, 14874–14884.

125. Murray, G.M. & Peck, C.C. (2007). Orofacial pain and jaw muscle activity: a new model. *J Oro Pain*, **21(4)**, 263–278; discussion 79–88.

126. Okeson, J.P. (2014). *Bell's Oral and Facial Pain*, 7th edn. Chicago, IL: Quintessence Publishing Co. Inc., xiii, 546 p.

127. de Leeuw, R., Boering, G., Stegenga, B. & de Bont, L.G. (1994). Clinical signs of TMJ osteoarthrosis and internal derangement 30 years after nonsurgical treatment. *J Oro Pain.* **8(1)**, 18–24.

128. Stohler, C.S. & Zarb, G.A. (1999). On the management of temporomandibular disorders: a plea for a low-tech, high-prudence therapeutic approach. *J Oro Pain*, **13(4)**, 255–261.

Chapter 15

129. Simons, D.G., Travell, J.G. & Simons, L.S. (1999). *Travell & Simons' Myofascial Pain and Dysfunction: The Trigger Point Manual*, 2nd edn. Baltimore, MD: Williams & Wilkins.

130. Okeson, J.P. (2014). *Bell's Oral and Facial Pain*, 7th edn. Chicago, IL: Quintessence Publishing Co. Inc., pp. 151–155.

131. de Leeuw, J.R. & Klasser, G.D. (2013). *Orofacial Pain: Guidelines for Assessment, Diagnosis and Management*. 5th edn. Chicago, IL: Quintessence Publishing Co, Inc., ix, 301 p.

132. Weiss, T.M., Atanasov, S. & Calhoun, K.H. (2005). The association of tongue scalloping with obstructive sleep apnea and related sleep pathology. *Otol Head Neck Surg.*, **133(6)**, 966–971.

133. Gronqvist, J., Haggman-Henrikson, B. & Eriksson, P.O. (2008). Impaired jaw function and eating difficulties in whiplash-associated disorders. *Swed Dent J.*, **32(4)**, 171–177.

134. de Wijer, A., de Leeuw, J.R., Steenks, M.H. & Bosman, F. (1996). Temporomandibular and cervical spine disorders. Self-reported signs and symptoms. *Spine*, **21(14)**, 1638–1646.

135. de Wijer, A., Steenks, M.H., de Leeuw, J.R., Bosman, F. & Helders, P.J. (1996). Symptoms of the cervical spine in temporomandibular and cervical spine disorders. *J Oral Rehab.*, **23(11)**, 742–750.

136. De Laat, A., Meuleman, H., Stevens, A. & Verbeke, G. (1998). Correlation between cervical spine and temporomandibular disorders. *Clin Oral Invest.*, **2(2)**, 54–7.

137. Kraus. S. (2007). Temporomandibular disorders, head and orofacial pain: cervical spine considerations. *Dent Clin N Am.*, **51(1)**, 161–193, vii.

138. Mannheimer, J.S. & Rosenthal, R.M. (1991). Acute and chronic postural abnormalities as related to craniofacial pain and temporomandibular disorders. *Dent Clin N Am.*, **35(1)**, 185–208.

139. Watson, D.H. & Drummond, P.D. (2012). Head pain referral during examination of the neck in migraine and tension-type headache. *Headache*, **52(8)**, 1226–1235.

140. Haldeman, S., Carroll, L. & Cassidy, J.D. (2010). Findings from the bone and joint decade 2000 to 2010 task force on neck pain and its associated disorders. *J Occup Environ Med.*, **52(4)**, 424–427.

Chapter 16

141. Fokkens, W.J., Lund, V.J., Mullol, J., Bachert, C., Alobid, I., *et al.* (2012). European position paper on rhinosinusitis and nasal polyps. *Rhinol Suppl.* **(23)**, 3 p. preceding table of contents, 1–298.

142. Schlosser, R. & Harvey, R. (2008). Diagnosis of chronic. In: *Rhinosinusitis* (eds E. Thaler & D.W. Kennedy), New York: Springer, pp. 1–24.

143. Tartaryn, R. (2008). Rhinosinusitis and endodontic disease. In: *Ingle's Endodontics*, 6th edn (ed. J Ingle), Hamilton, BC: Decker Inc., pp. 626–627.

144. Orlandi, R. (2008). Medical management of acute rhinosinusitis. In: *Rhinosinusitis* (eds E. Thaler & D.W. Kennedy), New York: Springer, pp. 1–10.

145. Wolff, H.G. (1963). *Headache and Other Head Pain*, 2nd edn. New York: Oxford University Press, 773 p.

146. Bhattacharyya, N. (2003). The economic burden and symptom manifestations of chronic rhinosinusitis. *Am J Rhinol.*, **17(1)**, 27–32.

147. Patel, N.A. & Ferguson, B.J. (2012). Odontogenic sinusitis: an ancient but under-appreciated cause of maxillary sinusitis. *Curr Op Otol Head Neck Surg.*, **20(1)**, 24–28.

148. Bomeli, S.R., Branstetter, B.F. & Ferguson, B.J. (2009). Frequency of a dental source for acute maxillary sinusitis. *Laryngoscope*, **119(3)**, 580–584.

149. Tomomatsu, N., Uzawa, N., Aragaki, T. & Harada, K. (2014). Aperture width of the osteomeatal complex as a predictor of successful treatment of odontogenic maxillary sinusitis. *Int J Oral Maxillofac Surg.*, **43(11)**, 1386–1390.

150. Legenth, F., Billet, J., Beauvillain, C., Bonnet, J. & Miegeville, M. (1989). The role of dental canal fillings in the development of Aspergillus sinusitis. A report of 85 cases. *Arch Otorhinolaryngol.*, **246(5)**, 318–320.

151. Nurbakhsh, B., Friedman, S., Kulkarni, G.V., Basrani, B. & Lam, E. (2011). Resolution of maxillary sinus mucositis after endodontic treatment of maxillary teeth with apical periodontitis: a cone-beam computed tomography pilot study. *J Endod.*, **37(11)**, 1504–1511.

152. Nair, U.P. & Nair, M.K. (2010). Maxillary sinusitis of odontogenic origin: cone-beam volumetric computerized tomography-aided diagnosis. *Oral Surg Oral Med Oral Path Oral Radio Endo.*, **110(6)**, e53–e57.

153. Bell, G.W., Joshi, B.B. & Macleod, R.I. (2011). Maxillary sinus disease: diagnosis and treatment. *Br Dent J.*, **210(3)**, 113–118.

154. Brook, I. (2006). Sinusitis of odontogenic origin. *Otol Head Neck Surg.*, **135(3)**, 349–355.

155. Longhini, A.B., Branstetter, B.F. & Ferguson, B.J. (2012). Otolaryngologists' perceptions of odontogenic maxillary sinusitis. *Laryngoscope*, **122(9)**, 1910–1914.

156. Longhini, A.B. & Ferguson, B.J. (2011). Clinical aspects of odontogenic maxillary sinusitis: a case series. *Int Forum Allerg Rhinol.*, **1(5)**, 409–415.

157. Low, K.M., Dula, K., Burgin, W. & von Arx, T. (2008). Comparison of periapical radiography and limited cone-beam tomography in posterior maxillary teeth referred for apical surgery. *J Endod.*, **34(5)**, 557–562.

158. Martines, F., Salvago, P., Ferrara, S., Mucia, M., Gambino, A. & Sireci, F. (2014). Parietal subdural empyema as complication of acute odontogenic sinusitis: a case report. *J Med Case Rep.*, **8**, 282.

159. Williams, J.W., Jr., Simel, D.L., Roberts, L. & Samsa, G.P. (1992). Clinical evaluation for sinusitis. Making the diagnosis by history and physical examination. *Ann Intern Med.*, **117(9)**, 705–710.

160. Chandra, R. (2008). Medical management of chronic rhinosinusitis. In: Rhinosinusitis (eds E. Thaler & D.W. Kennedy), New York: Springer, pp. 1–17.

161. Harvey, R., Hannan, S.A., Badia, L. & Scadding, G. (2007). Nasal saline irrigations for the symptoms of chronic rhinosinusitis. *Cochrane Database of Systematic Reviews*, **3**, CD006394.

162. Huang, W.H. & Fang, S.Y. (2004). High prevalence of antibiotic resistance in isolates from the middle meatus of children and adults with acute rhinosinusitis. *Am J Rhinol.*, **18(6)**, 387–391.

163. Abuzaid, W. & Thaler, E. (2008). Etiology and impact of rhinosinusitis. In: *Rhinosinusitis*: (eds E. Thaler & D.W. Kennedy), New York: Springer, pp. 1–15.

Chapter 17

164. Katsarava, Z. & Steiner, T.J. (2012). Neglected headache: ignorance, arrogance or insouciance? *Cephalalgia*, **32(14)**, 1019–1020.

165. Headache Classification Committee of the International Headache Society (2013). *The International Classification of Headache Disorders*, 3rd edn (beta version). *Cephalalgia*, **33(9)**, 629–808.

166. Lynch, K.M. & Brett, F. (2012). Headaches that kill: a retrospective study of incidence, etiology and clinical features in cases of sudden death. *Cephalalgia*, **32(13)**, 972–978.

167. Joubert, J. (2013). Diagnosing headache. *Aust Fam Physic.*, **34(8)**, 621–625.

168. Benoliel, R. & Eliav, E. (2013). Primary headache disorders. *Dent Clin N Am.*, **57(3)**, 513–539.

169. Kaniecki, R.G. (2012). Tension-type headache. *Continuum (Minneap Minn)*, **18(4)**, 823–834.

170. Schiffman, E., Ohrbach, R., List, T., Anderson, G., Jensen, R., et al. (2012). Diagnostic criteria for headache attributed to temporomandibular disorders. *Cephalalgia.* **32(9)**, 683–692.

171. Fumal, A. & Schoenen, J. (2008). Tension-type headache: current research and clinical management. *Lancet Neurol.*, **7(1)**:70–83.

172. Joubert, J. (2005). Migraine – diagnosis and treatment. *Aust Fam Physic.*, **34(8)**, 627–632.

173. Charles, A. (2012). Migraine is not primarily a vascular disorder. *Cephalalgia*, **32(5)**, 431–432.

174. Bruijn, J., Duivenvoorden, H., Passchier, J., Locher, H., Dijkstra, N. & Arts, W.F. (2010). Medium-dose riboflavin as a prophylactic agent in children with migraine: a preliminary placebo-controlled, randomised, double-blind, cross-over trial. *Cephalalgia*, **30(12)**, 1426–1434.

Chapter 18

175. Silberstein, S.D., Lipton, R.B., Dodick, D. & Wolff, H.G. (2008). Wolff's Headache and Other Head Pain, 8th edn (eds S.D. Silberstein, R.B. Lipton & D.W. Dodick), Oxford; New York: Oxford University Press, xx, 844 p.

176. Krabbe, A.A. (1986). Cluster headache: a review. *Acta Neurol Scand.*, **74(1)**, 1–9.

177. Russell, M.B. (2004). Epidemiology and genetics of cluster headache. *Lancet Neurol.*, **3(5)**, 279–283.

178. Fischera, M., Marziniak, M., Gralow, I. & Evers, S. (2008). The incidence and prevalence of cluster headache: a meta-analysis of population-based studies. *Cephalalgia*, **28(6)**, 614–618.

179. Headache Classification Subcommittee of the International Headache Society (2004). *The International Classification of Headache Disorders*, 2nd edn. *Cephalalgia*, **24(Suppl 1)**, 9–160.

180. Voiticovschi-Iosob, C., Allenam M., De Cillism I., Nappim G., Sjaastadm O. & Antonacim F. (2014). Diagnostic and therapeutic errors in cluster headache: a hospital-based study. *J Headache Pain*, **15**, 56.

181. Razvi, S.S., Walker, L., Teasdale, E., Tyagi, A. & Muir, K.W. (2006). Cluster headache due to internal carotid artery dissection. *J Neurol.*, **253(5)**, 661–663.

182. Antonaci, F. & Sjaastad, O. (1989). Chronic paroxysmal hemicrania (CPH): a review of the clinical manifestations. *Headache*, **29(10)**, 648–656.

183. Bahra, A., May, A. & Goadsby, P.J. (2002). Cluster headache: a prospective clinical study with diagnostic implications. *Neurology*, **58(3)**, 354–361.

Chapter 19

184. Love, S. & Coakham, H.B. (2001). Trigeminal neuralgia: pathology and pathogenesis. *Brain*, **124(12)**, 2347–2360.

185. Chen, G.Q., Wang, X.S., Wang, L. & Zheng, J.P. (2014). Arterial compression of nerve is the primary cause of trigeminal neuralgia. *Neurol Sci.*, **35(1)**, 61–66.

186. Jannetta, P.J. (1980). Neurovascular compression in cranial nerve and systemic disease. *Ann Surg.*, **192(4)**, 518–525.

187. Smith, J.H. & Cutrer, F.M. (2011). Numbness matters: a clinical review of trigeminal neuropathy. *Cephalalgia*, **31(10)**, 1131–1144.

188. Dworkin, S.I., Porrino, L.J. & Smith, J.E. (1992). Importance of behavioral controls in the analysis of ongoing events. *NIDA Res Monogr.*, **124**, 173–188.

189. Fromm, G.H., Graff-Radford, S.B., Terrence, C.F. & Sweet, W.H. (1990). Pre-trigeminal neuralgia. *Neurology*, **40(10)**, 1493–1495.

190. de Siqueira, S.R., Nobrega, J.C., Valle, L.B., Teixeira, M.J. & de Siqueira, J.T. (2004). Idiopathic trigeminal neuralgia: clinical aspects and dental procedures. *Oral Surg Oral Med Oral Pathol Oral Radiol Endod.*, **98(3)**, 311–315.

191. Broggi, G., Ferroli, P., Franzini, A., Servello, D. & Dones, I. (2000). Microvascular decompression for trigeminal neuralgia: comments on a series of 250 cases, including 10 patients with multiple sclerosis. *J Neurol Neurosurg Psych.*, **68(1)**, 59–64.

192. Parmar, M., Sharma, N., Modgill, V. & Naidu, P. (2013). Comparative evaluation of surgical procedures for trigeminal neuralgia. *J Maxillofac Oral Surg.*, **12(4)**, 400–409.

193. De Simone, R., Marano, E., Brescia Morra, V., Ranieri, A., Ripa, P., *et al.* (2005). A clinical comparison of trigeminal neuralgic pain in patients with and without underlying multiple sclerosis. *Neurol Sci.*, **26(Suppl 2)**, s150–s151.

Chapter 20

194. Balasubramaniam, R., Kuperstein, A.S. & Stoopler, E.T. (2014). Update on oral herpes virus infections. *Dent Clin N Am.*, **58(2)**, 265–280.
195. Woo, S.B. & Challacombe, S.J. (2007). Management of recurrent oral herpes simplex infections. *Oral Surg Oral Med Oral Pathol Oral Radiol Endod.*, **103(Suppl S12)**, e1–e8.
196. Nalamachu, S. & Morley-Forster, P. (2012). Diagnosing and managing postherpetic neuralgia. *Drugs Aging*, **29(11)**, 863–869.
197. Roxas, M. (2006). Herpes zoster and postherpetic neuralgia: diagnosis and therapeutic considerations. *Altern Med Rev.*, **11(2)**, 102–113.
198. Weaver, B.A. (2007). The burden of herpes zoster and postherpetic neuralgia in the United States. *J Am Osteopath Assoc.*, **107(3 Suppl 1)**, S2–S7.
199. Strommen, G.L., Pucino, F., Tight, R.R. & Beck, C.L. (1988). Human infection with herpes zoster: etiology, pathophysiology, diagnosis, clinical course, and treatment. *Pharmacotherapy*, **8(1)**, 52–68.
200. Fristad, I., Bardsen, A., Knudsen, G.C. & Molven, O. (2002). Prodromal herpes zoster–a diagnostic challenge in endodontics. *Int Endod J.*, **35(12)**, 1012–1016.
201. Patil, S., Srinivas, K., Reddy, B.S. & Gupta, M. (2013). Prodromal herpes zoster mimicking odontalgia – a diagnostic challenge. *Ethiop J Health Sci.*, **23(1)**, 73–77.
202. Heiman, J.L. (1972). Case report: odontalgia resulting from prodromal herpes zoster. *J Mich State Dent Assoc.*, **54(3)**, 102–105.
203. Goon, W.W. & Jacobsen, P.L. (1988). Prodromal odontalgia and multiple devitalized teeth caused by a herpes zoster infection of the trigeminal nerve: report of case. *J Am Dent Assoc.*, **116(4)**, 500–504.
204. Tidwell, E., Hutson, B., Burkhart, N., Gutmann, J.L. & Ellis, C.D. (1999). Herpes zoster of the trigeminal nerve third branch: a case report and review of the literature. *Int Endod J.*, **32(1)**, 61–66.
205. Amlie-Lefond, C., Mackin, G.A., Ferguson, M., Wright, R.R., Mahalingam, R. & Gilden, D.H. (1996). Another case of virologically confirmed zoster sine herpete, with electrophysiologic correlation. *J Neurovirol.*, **2(2)**, 136–138.
206. Dworkin, R.H., Gnann, J.W., Jr., Oaklander, A.L., Raja, S.N., Schmader, K.E. & Whitley, R.J. (2008). Diagnosis and assessment of pain associated with herpes zoster and postherpetic neuralgia. *J Pain*, **9(1 Suppl 1)**, S37–S44.
207. Shapiro, M., Kvern, B., Watson, P., Guenther, L., McElhaney, J. & McGeer, A. (2011). Update on herpes zoster vaccination: a family practitioner's guide. *Can Fam Physician*, **57(10)**, 1127–1131.
208. Sigurdsson, A. & Jacoway, J.R. (1995). Herpes zoster infection presenting as an acute pulpitis. *Oral Surg Oral Med Oral Pathol Oral Radiol Endod.*, **80(1)**, 92–95.
209. Wagner, G., Klinge, H. & Sachse, M.M. (2012). Ramsay Hunt syndrome. *J Dtsch Dermatol Ges.*, **10(4)**, 238–244.
210. Sweeney, C.J. & Gilden, D.H. (2001). Ramsay Hunt syndrome. *J Neurol Neurosurg Psychiatry*, **71(2)**, 149–154.
211. Ryu, E.W., Lee, H.Y., Lee, S.Y., Park, M.S. & Yeo, S.G. (2012). Clinical manifestations and prognosis of patients with Ramsay Hunt syndrome. *Am J Otolaryngol.*, **33(3)**, 313–318.
212. Ingle, J.I., Bakland, L.K., Baumgartner, J.C. & Ingle, J.I. (2008). *Ovid Technologies Inc. Ingle's Endodontics 6*. Hamilton, Ontario; Lewiston, NY: BC Decker, xxv, 1555 p.
213. Weaverg B.A. (2009). Herpes zoster overview: natural history and incidence. *J Am Osteopath Assoc.*, **109(6 Suppl 2)**, S2–S6.

214. Opstelten, W., Mauritz, J.W., de Wit, N.J., van Wijck, A.J., Stalman, W.A. & van Essen, G.A. (2002). Herpes zoster and postherpetic neuralgia: incidence and risk indicators using a general practice research database. *Fam Pract.*, **19(5)**, 471–475.
215. Argoff, C.E. (2011). Review of current guidelines on the care of post-herpetic neuralgia. *Postgrad Med.*, **123(5)**, 134–142.

Chapter 21

216. Kawasaki, A. & Purvin, V. (2009). Giant cell arteritis: an updated review. *Acta Ophthalmol.*, **87(1)**, 13–32.
217. Weyand, C.M. & Goronzy, J.J. (2014). Giant-cell arteritis and polymyalgia rheumatica. *N Engl J Med.*, **371(17)**, 1653.
218. Lee, A.G. (1995). A case report. Jaw claudication: a sign of giant cell arteritis. *J Am Dent Assoc.*, **126(7)**, 1028–1029.
219. Allen, D.T, Voytovich, M.C. & Allen, J.C. (2000). Painful chewing and blindness: signs and symptoms of temporal arteritis. *J Am Dent Assoc.*, **131(12)**, 1738–1741.
220. Goicochea, M., Correale, J., Bonamico, L., Dominguez, R., Bagg, E., *et al.* (2007). Tongue necrosis in temporal arteritis. *Headache*, **47(8)**, 1213–1215.
221. Llorente Pendas, S., De Vicente Rodriguez, J.C., Gonzalez Garcia, M., Junquera Gutierrez, L.M. & Lopez Arranz, J.S. (1994). Tongue necrosis as a complication of temporal arteritis. *Oral Surg Oral Med Oral Pathol.*, **78(4)**, 448–451.
222. Marcos, O., Cebrecos, A.I., Prieto, A. & Sancho de Salas, M. (1998). Tongue necrosis in a patient with temporal arteritis. *J Oral Maxillofac Surg.*, **56(10)**, 1203–1206.
223. Rockey, J.G. & Anand, R. (2002). Tongue necrosis secondary to temporal arteritis: a case report and literature review. *Oral Surg Oral Med Oral Pathol Oral Radiol Endod.*, **94(4)**, 471–473.
224. Maidana, D.E., Munoz, S., Acebes, X., Llatjos, R., Jucgla, A & Alvarez, A. (2011). Giant cell arteritis presenting as scalp necrosis. *Sci World J.*, **11**, 1313–1315.
225. Morris, O.C., Paine, M.A. & O'Day, J. (2006). Giant cell arteritis presenting with scalp necrosis – the timing of temporal artery biopsy? *Clin Experi Ophthalmol.*, **34(7)**, 715–716.
226. Adams, W.B. & Becknell, C.A. (2007). Rare manifestation of scalp necrosis in temporal arteritis. *Arch Dermatol.*, **143(8)**, 1079–1080.
227. Schievink, W.I. (2001). Spontaneous dissection of the carotid and vertebral arteries. *N Engl J Med.*, **344(12)**, 898–906.
228. Thanvi, B., Munshi, S.K., Dawson, S.L. & Robinson, T.G. (2005). Carotid and vertebral artery dissection syndromes. *Postgrad Med J.*, **81(956)**, 383–388.
229. Chan, C.C., Paine, M. & O'Day, J. (2001). Carotid dissection: a common cause of Horner's syndrome. *Clin Experi Ophthalmol.*, **29(6)**, 411–415.
230. Stence, N.V., Fenton, L.Z., Goldenberg, N.A., Armstrong-Wells, J. & Bernard T.J. (2011). Craniocervical arterial dissection in children: diagnosis and treatment. *Curr Treat Options Neurol.*, **13(6)**, 636–648.
231. Mokri, B., Silbert, P.L., Schievink, W.I. & Piepgras, D.G. (1996). Cranial nerve palsy in spontaneous dissection of the extracranial internal carotid artery. *Neurology*, **46(2)**, 356–359.

Chapter 22

232. Teodoro, F.C., Tronco, M.F., Jr., Zampronio, A.R., Martini, A.C., Rae, G.A. & Chichorro, J.G. (2013). Peripheral substance P and neurokinin-1 receptors have a role in inflammatory and neuropathic orofacial pain models. *Neuropeptides*, **47(3)**, 199–206.
233. Marbach, J.J. (1993). Is phantom tooth pain a deafferentation (neuropathic) syndrome? Part II: Psychosocial considerations. *Oral Surg Oral Med Oral Pathol.*, **75(2)**, 225–232.

234. Marbach, J.J. & Raphael, K.G. (2000). Phantom tooth pain: a new look at an old dilemma. *Pain Med.*, **1(1)**, 68–77.

235. Headache Classification Committee of the International Headache Society (2013). *The International Classification of Headache Disorders*, 3rd edn (beta version). *Cephalalgia*, **33(9)**, 629–808.

236. Hampf, G., Vikkula, J., Ylipaavalniemi, P. & Aalberg, V. (1987). Psychiatric disorders in orofacial dysaesthesia. *Int J Oral Maxillofac Surg.*, **16(4)**, 402–407.

237. Vickers, E.R., Boocock, H., Harris, R.D., Bradshaw, J., Cooper, M., *et al.* (2006). Analysis of the acute postoperative pain experience following oral surgery: identification of "unaffected", "disabled" and "depressed, anxious and disabled" patient clusters. *Aust Dent J.*, **51(1)**, 69–77.

238. Saarto, T. & Wiffen, P.J. (2010). Antidepressants for neuropathic pain: a Cochrane review. *J Neurol Neurosurg Psych.*, **81(12)**, 1372–1373.

239. Moore, A., Wiffen, P. & Kalso, E. (2014). Antiepileptic drugs for neuropathic pain and fibromyalgia. *JAMA*, **312(2)**, 182–183.

240. Moore, R.A., Wiffen, P.J., Derry, S., Toelle, T. & Rice, A.S. (2014). Gabapentin for chronic neuropathic pain and fibromyalgia in adults. *Cochrane Database Syst Rev.*, **4**, CD007938.

241. Vickers, E.R., Karsten, E., Flood, J. & Lilischkis, R. (2014). A preliminary report on stem cell therapy for neuropathic pain in humans. *J Pain Res.*, **7**, 255–263.

Chapter 23

242. Vickers, E.R., Boocock, H., Harris, R.D., Bradshaw, J., Cooper, M., *et al.* (2006). Analysis of the acute postoperative pain experience following oral surgery: identification of "unaffected", "disabled" and "depressed, anxious and disabled" patient clusters. *Aust Dent J.*, **51(1)**, 69–77.

Index

Page numbers in *italics* indicate figures; page numbers in **bold** indicate tables

Diagnosing Dental and Orofacial Pain: A Clinical Manual, First Edition. Edited by Alex J. Moule and M. Lamar Hicks.
© 2017 John Wiley & Sons, Ltd. Published 2017 by John Wiley & Sons, Ltd.
Companion website: www.wiley.com/go/moule/dental_and_orofacial_pain

Printed and bound by CPI Group (UK) Ltd, Croydon, CR0 4YY

21/06/2024

14518428-0001

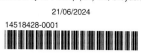